The Longest Farewell

To my darling James,
and to Bonnie and Phil – The Trinity.

The Longest Farewell

James, Dementia and Me

Nula Suchet

SEREN

Seren is the book imprint of
Poetry Wales Press Ltd,
57 Nolton Street, Bridgend, Wales, CF31 3AE

www.serenbooks.com
facebook.com / SerenBooks
Twitter: @SerenBooks

ISBN: 9781781725184
Ebook: 9781781725191

A CIP record for this title is available from the British Library.

The publisher acknowledges the financial assistance of the Welsh
Books Council.

Front cover image: James, before the onset of dementia, summer 1994
Back cover image: Trekking with John to Machu Picchu, spring 2018

Printed by Bell & Bain Ltd, Scotland

Contents

1. The Beginning 7

2. Something Feels Not Quite Right 11

3. Juggling while there's an Elephant in the Room 15

4. The Working James 19

5. James Retreating, while I'm in Denial 26

6. The Tipping Point – No More Denial 37

7. Diagnosis 43

8. Sucking the Sweetness 51

9. Getting Harder 58

10. Travels and the Difficulties of Out and About 67

11. Isolation 74

12. The Care Home Beckons 79

13. Listing the Last Times 83

14. Grief and Letting Go 89

15. Visiting Time 94

16. A Friend in Need 104

17. Tentative Steps 117

18. Uncertain Times 122

19. Like a Mistress, while a Wife 129

20. Sentenced to a Non-Life 143

21. Kinder to Animals 153

22. Final Goodbyes 168

23. Making a New Life 174

24. Postcript 177

Acknowledgements 181

1 : The Beginning

I loved you first: but afterwards your love
Outsoaring mine, sang such a loftier song...
— Christina Rosetti

My husband James is changing and I don't know why. Nor, if I'm absolutely honest, do I want to think about it because if I do I start to feel scared.

He's not himself.

I don't mean by that that he's feeling ill, it's just that he is not on top of things, and that is uncharacteristic. He isn't organising his work desk or bothering to tidy away things in the kitchen, which he's always done before – and, more unsettling, his personal hygiene has slipped. I'm constantly making allowances: maybe it's the odd-sock-wearing nutty professor coming out in him, a characteristic of the distracted creative – he's a writer, after all. That must be why he's forgetting to clean his teeth.

I'm doing my best to adapt to his strange moods and the odd things he does. I find myself brushing the starker facts under the carpet: he's stressed, there's too much on his plate, he's getting scatty in his old age.

But the thing is that James isn't very old: he's only

fifty-seven. Surely he shouldn't be losing his keys and glasses quite so often, or leaving his favourite jacket and valuable wristwatch on a film shoot, or his passport on a plane? And why is he forgetting to return important work calls? That I find really worrying. It's not like him at all. He lives and breathes his work, he's in it day and night, often compulsively, writing screenplays and documentary scripts about the subjects closest to his heart. James has enormous empathy for the struggling man and especially likes stories about people who have overcome huge challenges. I'm beginning to wonder: are we about to have challenges of our own to deal with?

But I'm not going to think about anything like that, at least, not yet. He's just stressed; it's a phase we'll have to get through, that's all.

* * *

It's hard to tell when the first signs of Pick's Disease, a particularly brutal form of dementia which affects the frontal lobes of the brain, started to show in James. But this is the beginning of what was to be the most terrifying and painful journey of both our lives. It's a condition that can affect men and women in their prime, like James, and there is no cure. Patients and their carers usually find themselves cast off by the medical profession – 'Sorry, there's nothing more we can do for you' – and adrift on an increasingly turbulent sea. That's how it was to be for us for eleven soul-destroying and utterly frightening years.

Just when things were becoming so bleak – once James was living in a care home – I found a friend whose wife Bonnie was in the same care home, also with early-onset dementia. John became my comfort, and for a couple of years there were four of us inextricably entwined in the strangest dance of love and care. It helped me so much to talk to someone who was experiencing so many of the same things.

At some point during James's life in the care home I wrote a memoir of what had been happening to us both, which came out in a torrent of words on the page. It was only later that I organised it and added a few short commentary paragraphs, tempered by the benefit of hindsight.

At the beginning I was full of incomprehension. How could this be happening to James, of all people? He had always been a brilliant man, talented and bright-eyed, with a wealth of emotional intelligence. How could this quicksilver, funny, logical and sensitive mind be attacked in this way?

* * *

James was born and brought up in Belfast in a very loving family. He passed his eleven plus and moved on to grammar school, and from there he went to London where he graduated with a degree in Economics and Politics from the London School of Economics. But he wanted a career in television as a cameraman.

As a young lad in the streets around the Falls Road, he had watched the BBC camera crews filming the Troubles in Belfast. It triggered in him a huge fascination with the whole process of telling a story to camera. After the LSE he got a job as a researcher with the BBC, before applying to train as a cameraman. He competed with over a thousand applicants and was thrilled when he was accepted for the prestigious course. He would go on to win many awards for his camera work, on programmes like Panorama, Z Cars, Play of the Week and on many documentaries, before graduating to writing and directing his own programmes.

2 : Something Feels Not Quite Right

For standing in your heart,
Is where I want to be, and long to be;
Ah, but I may as well try and catch the wind.
— *Donovan*

James has lost all interest in cooking. I can't remember the last time he made one of his Indian curries. When he's not filming and I'm working, he always does the food shopping and cooks the evening meal for my return. He spends hours choosing the spices to marinate the meat, and his food is beyond delicious.

Now it feels like an age since I last came back to a steamy kitchen, redolent with the smell of spice – so warm and welcoming with Lucy and Spanny, our two dogs, milling around his feet while he moves happily about.

Kathleen, a local girl who comes in four hours a week to help with the housework, has noticed things are different with James.

'I don't think James is himself. There's something not right. It's not like him to leave all the dirty dishes piled up in the sink,' she tells me worriedly. 'And he's leaving food uncovered. Not putting it away in the fridge anymore.'

This is not James.

Around this time, I take James to the doctor. He's been complaining of a pain down his left leg and is having difficulty passing water. This isn't the first time I've tried to have it checked out but in both cases the tests have come back negative.

This doctor is a family friend. He listens as we tell him the symptoms, then concludes that it's just a case of James being neurotic and possibly suffering from mild depression.

He gives his diagnosis, smiling. 'James, I can find nothing wrong with you. I suggest you get out of the house, stop writing and get into the real world. Get back to directing and mixing with people. Earn some money.'

I'm annoyed by the doctor's unsympathetic attitude. But one thing is true, James hasn't been getting out, and all he seems to want to do is closet himself away to write. And never mind earning money – James is no longer paying the bills. He's leaving them unopened, not from any fear that we haven't the money to pay them, but due to this new and growing incapacity that steals daily over his life.

Our home is in a very rural part of the country. With no nearby neighbours we are isolated. With James not earning money I'm beginning to feel stressed about the cost of maintaining such a large house. Maybe we should move closer to Dublin. James would have the stimulus he needs, I reasoned, to bring him out of himself. He could get out and about and mix with people.

* * *

We decide to go away for the weekend. I have the perfect place – a salmon fishing lake we both love in County Kerry – where we can chat about the future and make a plan.

We stay in a country house we know well, perched on the shores of the lake. James's passion for fly fishing had been ignited some years before whilst making a documentary on the salmon fishing of Scotland, when he had been lucky to have Prince Charles's ghillie as his tutor. Although I don't fish I love going out with him. I take my sketch pad and position myself further along the bank; we enjoy a quiet and peaceful companionship, the dogs milling about the lake shore, whiling away the hours until lunchtime when we share our picnic together.

Today I feel so happy, at one with nature and with James. It is an idyllic day, and not a cloud spoils our enjoyment of it. It's as if our recent troubles belong to other people, not to us.

There is a ripple, though. It breaks the halcyon perfection of the day later on, after we have packed up the fishing gear and picnic basket and returned to the house, content and hungry for supper. Always before when we've stayed here, after a delicious dinner cooked by a superb chef, James would join in with a group of local musicians, accompanying them on the piano. This evening, James insists he wants to go out fishing again. I cannot persuade him not to go back to the lake and I'm disappointed and a little confused. He promises he won't be too long.

It is midnight and there's no sign of James. I'm sitting in bed, trying not to worry. He'll appear any moment now, I reassure myself. By three in the morning I am feeling frantic and call the desk porter. I'm fearing the worst: the area round the lake is boggy and there's no lighting. What if James has fallen into the lake and drowned?

The desk porter is equally concerned and says he will call the police to send out a search party. I feel a strange conflict of emotions at his words – panic at what might have happened, coupled with a crossness with James that he had ever chosen to go out at all.

At that moment he walks in casually, smiling. He seems to have no concept that I might have been worried, and doesn't apologise, can't work out why I might have been concerned – a stance that kindles my anger into fury.

3 : Juggling while there's an Elephant in the Room

And I woke and found me here,
On the cold hill's side
— John Keats

Before James's diagnosis I would experience moments of anger or hot irritation, which I felt worse about after I knew that James's mind was in the grip of Picks Disease, the 'bastard dementia' as I called it. After diagnosis I became better at drawing from a wellspring of patience, although I didn't, by any means, manage to quench all the blazes of frustration that boiled up. I realised, on seeing how calm and efficient many of James's carers were later on, that in many ways it is much harder to care for someone whom you are closer to.

These early frustrations, and not a little fear, were partly caused by the 'other half' of the well-oiled machine that is good coupledom breaking down. Help! Where's my other half? Who can I call now to fix my computer glitch, telephone me when I'm on a long journey to make sure I've stopped for a coffee and something to eat, feed the dogs when I'm late back from work, meet me at the airport after a work trip?

One of the lovely things about being a mutually supportive couple is that you're there for each other, you're thinking about each other wherever you may be. The loneliness of arriving, unmet, at a station platform at night, or not seeing a smiling face at the arrivals hall and having to make your solitary way home, is one of those things that losing a partner brings home to you. But for now, James is still with me, and for the time being our life together is functioning with a scattering of odd glitches, and a degree of frustration and fury on my uncomprehending part!

I'm working so hard at the moment that I can hardly keep all the balls in the air, trying to keep my own design business running while constantly having to dive for the balls James seems continuously to be dropping. It's hard to lose the support and efficiency of your other half – my better half, I've always considered him. The hard fact is that for quite some time now all the earning is being done by me, as well as the major share of the household chores. James seems unconcerned that we have a large country house to maintain – it's as though money has ceased to mean anything to him – and the things he would always do to support me are dropping away.

Little things that cause a ripple of concern are multiplying daily. Only a few weeks after our fishing weekend I come back to the house in the evening after work to find the dogs biting at my ankles, desperate for food, and their water bowl dry. James dotes on Spanny, a Corgi, and Lucy, a Jack Russell, which makes his ignoring their needs so oddly uncharacteristic. He boasts about Spanny's exceptional talent at howling in unison to opera arias, and he is always very protective of Lucy, my little stray whom James nursed back to health after we found her on the roadside, emaciated and starving, some years ago.

Our previously tight ship feels as if it is listing badly, and I have the uneasy feeling – which borders on stark fear at times – that our helmsman is elsewhere while our leaky vessel is drifting out to sea.

* * *

It's late, the weather is grim, and I'm on the last plane to Dublin after an exhausting day in London visiting a client, whose design for renovating the interior of their large house in Eaton Square is finally complete. Take-off was delayed due to snowstorms, but I comforted myself that, despite the late hour, James will be waiting for me at the airport. It is always a huge joy and relief to see his face at the end of a long day, especially when I'm bone tired and longing to get home to a warm kitchen, welcoming dogs, some hot food, and a cuddle in front of the fire.

We disembark at midnight, but in the arrivals hall at Dublin airport there's no sign of James. Worried that he might have had an accident in the blizzard, I call home. I'm relieved when he picks up, but this turns into angry frustration when he cannot explain why he isn't here to meet me. From what I can gather, he's already been to the airport and, when my flight hadn't come in at the scheduled time, didn't hang around to wait for it and returned home.

Our house is two hours from the airport and, as I wait for James to pick me up, I'm feeling cold, exhausted and increasingly furious. It'll be four in the morning before I get home.

When he finally arrives at the airport I shout at him. 'James, why the hell didn't you wait for my flight? Why didn't you ask at the information desk? They'd have told you it'd been delayed.'

He doesn't answer and offers no explanation, merely picks up my bag and heads for the car. On the drive home he offers no apology and I don't speak to him for the rest of the journey.

The next day I raise it with him again, still confused at what happened the previous night. 'It's not like you not to have waited,' I tell him. 'You could have had a coffee and read the paper.'

He just looks at me blankly and appears not to know what I'm talking about.

I'm confused and don't know what to make of it, but then I put it aside and forget about it for the moment, too busy, keeping all those balls in the air, to do anything else.

4 : The Working James

But one man loved the pilgrim soul in you,
And loved the sorrows of your changing face.
— W.B. Yeats

For our entire married life I've been used to hearing James tapping away on his computer, often in the very early morning, which is his most creative time. He's always included me in his work, talking through his ideas, discussing how his screenplays should be made, and accepting my suggestions for a character or a situation that differed to him. I've loved being part of his world; from the moment we got together I've been in creative heaven. I watched him writing and making his dramas. When he travelled away to film for weeks at a time I'd fly out and join him, be it in America or Europe.

We worked on many projects together. One such story was the life of Dr Noel Browne, a man who against the odds of a tragically impoverished Irish background qualified as a doctor. Whilst doing an internship in England, Browne was inspired by the newly formed National Health Service. Returning to Ireland, he entered politics, was elected to the Dáil, and rose to the position of Minister for Health.

He tried to introduce The Mother and Child scheme into the Catholic dominated Ireland of the fifties, where money dictated your chances of getting medical attention, but came up against huge opposition from the head of the church, Archbishop McQuaid. James felt certain Noel Browne's story needed to be told on the big screen, and he and I spent hours researching and interviewing him.

After approaching the Irish Film Board, James was commissioned to write the screenplay and make the film. At the same time he was developing other projects. One told the story of the abduction of two young girls by two men who were on a murder spree. We obtained all the forensic details from a coroner and James was working hard on developing the screenplay.

Now, though, unlike before, there seems to be something frenetic about his writing. I wake in the middle of the night to find him hunched over his computer at 2am, typing away furiously at his keyboard. I cannot persuade him to come back to bed. He's written seven screenplays in a matter of months. Suddenly it's as if his life depends on them and it's as if he is aware that there's only a limited span of time in which he can get it all down. He has so much to say, so much he wants to write, so many half-finished projects, ideas that are jostling in his head.

James has always juggled several projects in the hope of getting one of them made. I've frequently marvelled at his ability to write screenplays in tandem while he waited for scripts to be accepted for development. Television and film boards commissioned him to write and make dramas. He produced and directed several, with titles like Elizabeth Gaskell, The Love Series, and Trading Places.

He was an extraordinary human being. He cared so much about the inequalities of his fellow man. He wanted everyone to have a fair chance in life. He detested the large corporations where only profit mattered. Now there seems to be less and less of the deft and efficient juggler; he can't even get it together to answer calls, and shows no sign of wanting to direct any more.

I wish he didn't look so desperate and lonely sitting hunched over his desk, tapping away at the keyboard as if there's a hound from hell biting at his heels and his time is running out.

Natalie, his secretary, is worried too, and for the first time brings her concerns to me. She's worked loyally for James for ten years, and no doubt she's been keeping her concerns to herself for a while.

She says that James asked her to do some research, but his instructions made no sense, so she went back to him and queried them. He insisted it was okay, that's what he had meant, but on probing them further she became even more confused. He continued to insist angrily that his notes made sense, but she was adamant she could not decipher them.

'I think there's something strange going on,' she says.

I push her words aside. 'It's just James. He's a bit quirky.'

Two years ago James and I went to Prague to research the six-part series he was writing on Mozart. It was a happy time, James was excited and animated as he searched for all the sites related to his musical hero's life.

After that trip, Sony promised to fund the project, with American, Canadian and French networks also coming on board, following a series of very positive meetings. Back then it looked – as much as these things can look in the world of TV and film production – as if the series would go ahead and be made. It was an exciting time, as this, of all his work, was the closest to James's heart.

Two years on, having been told that Prague will be a much more cost-effective location than Vienna in which to film the series, we return to the city to do another recce.

This time James is distracted, no longer the sparky-eyed enthusiast he'd been that last time we'd been in Prague. It is as if he is just a shell of the old James, walking about aimlessly, not seeming to know what he needed to do. In the four days we are there we achieve nothing.

We return to Dublin and no more is said of the project. James ignores all further calls from Sony.

* * *

James and I fly to London for a meeting with a producer he has worked with before. David has read James's latest script, a comedy about a student who becomes a sperm donor to raise money for a trip on a Harley Davidson along Route 66. With a major film company interested, he is excited about its commercial potential.

He leans back in his chair, looks at James and says, 'Tell me more. How do you see it? Who do you see playing the characters?'

I wait for James to burst out with all kinds of ideas for the film. We have spent weeks talking into the night about the script. We hunted endlessly through Spotlight to find the perfect actors to play the characters in his story.

But James doesn't respond. He sits in silence. So David tries another question, then another and another. It's as if a strange language has been spoken, one James doesn't understand.

Now I'm confused, and embarrassed too. This isn't the James I know. Normally he wouldn't have stopped talking for a second; it would have been impossible to get a word in edgeways. Like David, I was waiting for him to describe his ideas for the storyline, locations and casting – every aspect of how his film should be made.

I ask him, 'What's the matter?' but he doesn't seem to understand the question.

What the hell is going on? Is he joking? We've flown all the way to London for this. It's an amazing opportunity. Now what?!

David turns to me, bewildered. 'Is there something wrong? Is James feeling all right?' Then he gives a laugh. 'Is he on something?'

I shrug my shoulders wordlessly, then try to fill in the gaps as far as I can with what I know, but this isn't my gig. I'm not James.

Now David moves past bewilderment to frustration, and then irritation. 'James, what the hell is going on? Why did you call this meeting?' He stands up, walks around his desk and stands over James. 'What the fuck is going on? Are you okay? I want to make this film but so far you've not uttered a word!'

James makes a few sounds, that make no sense. He doesn't try to apologise or explain why he hasn't responded or even why he's here.

'Fuck it, James. I love the script but I don't know what the fuck is going on with you.'

I stand up, flushed and embarrassed. 'I'm so sorry, David. When James gets his head together we'll come back and see you.'

I take James's arm and usher him to the door. He follows obediently without uttering a word. It is as if he doesn't know why he's here.

Outside the building, I lose it. 'What was all that about? What's going on? Why didn't you say something? Why didn't you tell him all those ideas you've had and the weeks you've spent rewriting and talking to me about it?' I rage on and on, repeating myself over and over again.

During my tirade of 'whys' James doesn't utter a word.

Instead, his lips move as if he's trying to say something, but no words come out. He appears to be in another world, somewhere else in his mind, and can't connect with me or anyone else.

We return home in silence.

5 : James Retreating, while I'm in Denial

Though nothing can bring back the hour
Of splendour in the grass, of glory in the flower.
– William Wordsworth

All those metaphors about denial are true for me. The elephant in the room certainly. The unflappable swan on the surface, whilst under the water the webbed feet are going like the clappers – for sure. I was the juggler wildly trying not to drop balls while Rome burns: how's that for a mixed metaphor!

I just didn't want to face up to what was going on. And anyway, I was running a thriving interior design practice with all that that entails, travelling, and dealing with clients whose lives bore no resemblance to my now chaotic private life. I'm so busy – paying bills, keeping us afloat – that I hardly had any energy left to work things out, never mind 'me' time. Maybe if I'd had some I might have worked through what was going on sooner. It's hard to do anything about something you really don't want to be happening at all. So I hid my head in the sand, and for the moment life went on in its rickety old way.

It's like some strange alien has entered our lives and it's spiralling out of control. James is retreating further and further into himself. I seem to be losing bits of him every day.

We go to a restaurant with my family to celebrate my sister's birthday. Everyone's happily enjoying themselves when suddenly James stands up and, without a word, leaves the restaurant. I can see my family looking at each other, wondering if it was something someone said. They think his leaving was so abrupt he must have been offended by the conversation round the table.

I follow James outside and ask, 'Are you okay?'

He doesn't answer but walks to our car and stands there, indicating he wants to go home.

I excuse us and we leave.

It's strange because the normal filter that prevents our doing anything too embarrassing in public seems sometimes to have stopped working in James. This previously sensitive, caring, polite and thoughtful man is displaying some strange mood swings. Not only is his social functioning becoming less adept and dependable – so that it can, at times, seem as if he's behaving rudely – but his recent bouts of crying seem to be becoming more frequent.

I'm not one of those women who subscribe to the 'big boys don't cry' school of thought, but it's strange and unsettling when James's face is suddenly suffused with tears – not the moist-eyed sort where one can dab at the corners of the eyes, but a great big sobbing flood. Not only has James never been one to do this, but the crying comes at odd times, for no apparent reason.

The first time it happens, other than listening to opera or watching a sad film, James interrupts me to tell me he's just seen his grandmother. 'Where,' I ask. 'In the shrubs,' he replies, pointing to the bottom of the garden. He cries like a baby as he describes Granny Black in great detail. 'I miss her so much,' he stutters through his sobs.

James was eleven when Granny Black died, and he has never spoken of her much with me, although I know she adored her firstborn grandson and he was very fond of her. Now, as the floodgates open, the memories pour out – including how she, with a European background, introduced him to classical music and took him to see the great Italian tenor Gigli at a concert hall in Belfast. James speaks of her in the present tense, which adds to the strangeness of the episode.

Once again, I put the oddness of his behaviour down to his spending far too much time writing alone.

He's socialising less and less, retreating more and more into his silent world. I want to cry out, 'Where is the bright, articulate, animated and capable man I know? Who is this strange new James who seems unable to finish a sentence and can only cope with the most basic conversation?'

His old friends, Rod and Pete, have become tired of

waiting for James to return their calls and insist on meeting him. They tell me how oddly withdrawn he seems when they finally get together, how indifferent he is to the news of the day. I can see why they are confused: ordinarily, James is a complete news junkie who relishes events and is always the first to relay and debate the breaking news of the day, be it politics or celebrity gossip. So long as it is a good story it always has his attention. But it hasn't been like that for a while now.

Pete reminded me how, after Tony Blair had won the election in 1997, he and James stayed up all night to hear the results. I smile, remembering how ecstatic James had been at Labour's victory.

I try to put Pete's mind at rest but alarm bells go off in my head, as they do, intermittently, most days now. It's not only outsiders that James is becoming reluctant to communicate with, it's me too, and that's what is scaring me most.

* * *

I am invited to do some artwork for a television wildlife programme. I cannot believe my luck: I'll get to go to Tanzania, Zanzibar and the Seychelles. I need to get away, have a break from the endless worrying about James, and I'll get paid too, which makes it good on all fronts.

When I get there I find that while it is a welcome relief

and a distraction, the trip is tinged with sadness. It is overshadowed by the knowledge that I almost certainly won't be able to share the wonderful experience with James, tell him what I've been doing. Africa, and its hot sun over a red soil, brings back our shared past in waves.

Africa holds such a special place in our hearts. It is where we met, two decades before, when I was the artist commissioned to create drawings and sculptures for Ape Man, a four-part documentary series on Early Man that James was directing. We'd been working in Kenya and Tanzania then, too, and I'd fallen in love with the vibrant, funny, brilliant James.

Five years before I had liberated myself from an unhappy marriage, which had come on the heels of a difficult childhood in which I had felt frozen out by an unloving mother. Now I felt myself unfurl and start to flourish in the warmth of the African sun as we camped in a little township in the Rift Valley, south-west of Nairobi.

Each day James directed me as I sculpted fertility symbols of naked women with huge breasts and buttocks from the red clay. These lucky mascots were used by Early Man to ensure women would produce many offspring.

Filming took place in Magadi, a small township south-west of Nairobi. Here the terrain resembled early life in Africa, unchanged for thousands of years. The location was perfect for the series and overwhelmed me with its drama. The film crew set up on the shores of Lake Magadi, the southern-most lake in the Kenyan Rift Valley. Its exotic inhabitants, thousands of pink flamingoes, added to the sense of theatre. We lived amongst the Masai tribe, who had lived and worked here for centuries, and who were still dressed in their traditional red garments.

After the day's filming, the crew dined under a gorgeous star-staged sky, our table lit by Tilley lamps, which gave a lustre to the evening, and added to the romance of it all. As I sat surrounded by the sounds of Africa, I listened to the most riveting conversation by the wonderful minds around the table, hired for their expertise in Early Man. They discussed and debated evolution, Early Man's art, tools, survival and religion.

Walter Cronkite, America's most respected broadcaster journalist, who announced President Kennedy's death in 1963, was the narrator of the series and amused us with his tales of the shenanigans of American government leaders and celebrities. I was in my element, and entranced.

Often, during these dinners, James too entertained us with stories of his filming days for the BBC, Granada and A&E Television, and the characters he'd worked with. I sat there enthralled. In the six weeks of filming I became more and more drawn to the tall and handsome director, and his beautiful way of thinking and talking. He had striking green eyes that shone with enthusiasm, and spoke with the softest hint of a cultured Northern Irish accent. He was so secure in his own skin, totally confident, and completely unaware of his good looks.

He asked about my family and my past. We discovered that we shared many things, not least that we were both from Ireland and missed the country of our roots. Added to that we had both spent many years with the wrong person, but again – another similarity – we had both extricated ourselves and were now single.

I didn't think for a moment that James had singled me out in any special way. However, filming needed to continue once we returned to England. In the Chislehurst caves I needed to make drawings similar to those done by early man, such as six-foot bison.

James directed me while filming took place, and slowly it became obvious that our connection was deepening. On the final day, as we left the set, James walked over and invited me out to dinner.

A few weeks later we met in a little restaurant and we couldn't stop talking, talking, talking. We shared a love of life, literature, films and writing. Outside the restaurant he kissed me. We were locked in an embrace for so long that people started to gather and laughingly cheer us on. I felt an enormous surge of pleasure I had never felt before. I had fallen in love. I knew I would never be able to let go. James called our meeting 'bashert' – Yiddish for a being together that was meant to be. For our next date, he invited me to a poetry reading evening where he asked Seamus Heaney to sign his new poetry collection for me.

It was only after meeting James that I realised what love really meant. A few weeks later he proposed to me, and on a cold November day, we married. I wore a red coat, red being my lucky colour. The Registrar, a priest named Father Pat Buckley, and a stranger, were our only attendees. The stranger played 'Plaisir d 'Amour' on an old piano, as we signed the register. We laughed at the ridiculousness of it all, when suddenly James leaned over to me and whispered, 'I will treasure and love you for the rest of my life, my darling Nula.' It was the happiest day of my entire life.

All of this comes back to me in a great flood of memories now that I'm back in Africa, though this time without James. I find nostalgia – invariably a benign emotion before now – has the power to probe sore and tender places that have arisen in my heart.

* * *

Things come to a head on a weekend away in the West of Ireland. It's becoming increasingly difficult to explain away James's strange behaviour, although I do my best to carry on as normal, albeit with my head in the sand.

This time it's our friend Rita, who practised as a doctor in a top New York hospital before coming to Ireland to retire, who tells me squarely, but kindly, that she thinks something is not quite right with James.

Over dinner she tries to engage James in conversation.

'James, what are you working on at the moment?' He doesn't appear to understand her question. 'What was your all-time favourite film?'

He's embarrassed as he struggles to make sense of her question and becomes incoherent, moving his hands in a sharp gesture that knocks his wine glass over. He is oblivious to the red wine spreading in a deep stain over her antique tablecloth and makes no apology for it.

Later Rita tells me, 'I think there's something not right with James. He's not been reacting normally to my questions and he seems very remote.' She suggests that I take him to see a specialist. 'I feel you should do it sooner rather than later,' she adds.

'Do you think it might be stress?'

'No,' she replied cautiously. 'I think it's more than that. Maybe something relating to his brain. A tumour perhaps, or a cognitive problem. Or maybe an internal bleed. You really do need to get it checked out.'

* * *

I'm still doing my best not to accept that anything is seriously wrong. Surely it makes sense that stress has caused James's forgetfulness and uncommunicative, withdrawn behaviour? After all, he has always been under pressure: directing is a stressful occupation, dealing with crews, producers, actors and editors, and waiting for financiers to come up with the money.

Added to this, television is changing. No more can you nip into a controller's office and flag an idea and get all the support to develop it. The whole process of getting a programme commissioned has become more complicated – with numerous meetings and layer upon layer of executive decision-making before any final commitment to make it is made.

James has no choice but to change direction, to write and develop his own scripts with his own producers. It's a nerve-wracking game. No wonder the mental overload has caused his brain to shut down for a while.

But then I swing back to the harsh realisation that there is surely something more. James thrives on challenges and loves his job too much for it to affect him that seriously. I wonder about the brain tumour: maybe Rita is right.

Anyway I'm sure, whatever it is, that it can be put right. James is indestructible and it will surely be sorted out.

It is a while before I take Rita's advice and seek help. In the meantime we have Christmas to get through, and a very busy time with my work, but as I will very soon find out, things are fast coming to a head.

6 : The Tipping Point
– No More Denial

Seems lak to me the sun done loss his light,
Seems lak to me der's nothin' goin' right
Sence you went away.

— *James Weldon Johnson*

I'm sitting on a plane to Boston looking out of the window, my shoulder turned away from James who is sitting beside me, a look of relaxed contentment on his face. To outsiders the scene must look completely normal: a happy couple setting out on their Christmas holiday break. The truth is, though, I'm not really looking out of that round porthole – I'm totally and utterly in shock, and for me it promises to be anything but a happy Christmas.

Four hours ago – a couple of hours before dawn – I was digging a grave in the dark, James by my side holding the torch. When I was done I put down the spade and knelt next to the cardboard box in which I'd laid my little Lucy, wrapped in one of my old cardigans, and her dog toys. I took a moment to cut a piece of fur from her coat, which I slipped into my pocket. I was shaking and traumatised, unable to bear the idea of laying her in the cold earth. All the while, beside me, James just stood like a statue, emotionless and silent.

I loved her so much. She was my first ever dog. She was devoted to me and I to her. Incredibly she would hear my car coming from a mile away and be waiting at the gate for me when I came home. James would often tell me when I had to work away, 'Lucy charges up to your bedroom every morning to greet you and when you're not there she returns crestfallen.' When I left to go to work she would sit, with the saddest face, at the front door. Sometimes, when I could, I would take her with me in the car. She loved that, and would visibly smile, showing her doggy teeth and leap with joy and excitement into the passenger seat of my car.

The thing I cannot get over now is that while I feel so bereft, knowing there'll be no little tail wagging for me when I get home, James seems to feel nothing at all. It adds to my feeling of incomprehension and pain: that he can have done what he did and sit here smiling as if it had never happened, as if he'd had no part in Lucy's death.

It had happened the previous afternoon. James had driven me to the hairdresser's in the village, as I had an important client house-warming dinner party later and needed to look my best. It was a nightmare trying to find a parking space so I asked him to pick me up an hour later. When we pulled into the drive afterwards the inconceivable thing happened.

Lucy and Spanny would always lie nonchalantly by the gate waiting for our return, and we'd always slow down to give them time to get up and out of the way. This time, though, James approached the drive unusually fast.

I shouted at him, 'For fuck's sake, slow down! Slow down! Slow down!'

It all happened so fast. I'll never forget Lucy's loud yelping cries. I jumped out of the car to find her lying on her back struggling, unable to get up.

I think the vet and his wife, who kindly drove home with me after Lucy had been put down, must have thought James's behaviour strange and unaccountable, as he looked on like an innocent child while we placed Lucy in her basket and covered her in her favourite rug. He stood in silence, seemingly having no understanding of what had happened, no idea of his part in Lucy's accident nor that he was in any way responsible. They must have presumed he was in shock.

I had no choice but to go to the party. They were wonderful clients whom I had worked with for many years and their newly restored home was their dream come true. It was pure agony trying to paste on a smile for the event; with the added Christmas cheer, everyone was laughing, drinking, and having fun.

I left as soon as I could and sobbed all the way home. James was awake when I got back, but he still said nothing about what had happened earlier. What was really strange was that not only was there no apology but he didn't seem to feel sad. Instead, after I got into bed beside him, he went straight to sleep. I lay awake all night, not understanding what the hell was going on.

We have a stopover in Boston. Here as I watch the families in our hotel coming and going, greeting each other with hugs and kisses, I feel desperate. My sense of confusion and isolation is made worse by their excited laughter and chatter, festive with Christmas spirit, while I sit in raw turmoil with my silent partner, unable to understand what is going on with our life and where it is taking us. So I drink to deaden the sadness and hope things will feel better in Florida.

* * *

We're here in the haven of our house next to the creek, with its deck surrounded by water and mangroves. For once, though, it isn't giving me the restorative balm it usually offers when we hole up snugly to watch films and read books, happy that we've escaped the Christmas rush that sends the rest of the world into a mad spin. The pain of losing Lucy pervades my thoughts, but it's not just that. There is an awareness of cracks in our life, which fractures the calm, and there's a constant hum of fear in me, a feeling in the pit of my stomach that won't go away.

My sister and her husband have a home not far from

ours. As usual they invite us onto their boat for what has become a ritual Christmas Eve event, with other members of their family, down from New York, joining us.

It is a beautiful day out on the bay and we have the added joy of watching the dolphins follow our boat as the sun goes down. The sunsets in the Gulf of Mexico are extraordinarily lovely and I always feel blessed when we're out on the water. We moor near the shore and from there it's a short swim to the beach of the sumptuous Ritz Carlton where, as in previous years, we plan to have one of their famous pina coladas.

As Iori, my Welsh brother-in-law, puts down the anchor everyone lines up to jump off the boat and swim the short distance to shore. They all know I'm a poor swimmer and will never swim out of my depth, having almost drowned some years before in the Sea of Galilee. My family is used to James, ever protective, swimming with me on his back. This is what he's done every time before, so they don't hesitate to dive from the stern of the boat and make for the beach themselves.

James has my best sunglasses, which I lent him earlier, and he dives into the water wearing them. Then, instead of making his way to the side of the boat to carry me ashore, he sets off without a backward glance. The others are all on the beach by now and they laugh, thinking it's a joke – that he's only pretending to leave me behind – but when he doesn't swim back to fetch me their laughter morphs into confused silence.

By the time Iori swims back to get me my embarrassment has turned to anger. What does James think he's doing? All I can feel when I finally get to the beach is that the day has been spoilt. I'm cross, and made even crosser when I find out James has lost my sunglasses and he makes no apology for having done so.

It is the first time that my family realise that something strange is going on.

On Christmas Day there's no present or card from James.

Usually he writes something beautiful. I've kept all his cards, with their delicate drawings and poetic words, written especially for me. His use and knowledge of language has always been sublime. He's a wordsmith who can quote any poem or reel off lines from books.

Days later in his drawer, I find sheets of paper and a card where he's attempted to write me a Christmas greeting, full of scribbles and crossings out.

'… and in everyday I am making you happy in every way I can …'

'I am loving you my darling Nuli and always to your loving embrace forever my

 Nuli …'

'And making you happy for ever.'

'Love my Nuli every darling, is me.

It goes on and on, scribbled and crossed out and

rewritten over and over again. I don't know what to make of it and put it down to his being stressed, the excuse I've been making for his behaviour for the last year.

Later, I realise that this was his last desperate attempt to write me a loving message, and it would be the last thing he ever wrote to me.

7 : Diagnosis

I do not know where either of us can turn – Louise Bogan

There was, I found, an extraordinary difference in how far medical professionals are able to empathise, and even how they handle the shocked patient and their family, professionally. When you first get a bleak or terminal diagnosis the shock is immense, the words don't sink in. Some doctors show tact, delicacy, understanding; others seem to barricade themselves against the emotion emanating from their client with a brusque outer shell, an armour of technical words, and even unimaginable tactlessness.

As for the patient or carer, some perhaps are able to take the news on board with stoical acceptance, but it wasn't so for me. James was like the innocent lamb; I was a barely contained Fury – and remained that way on and off, as I raged at the dying of James's light.

* * *

Finally I take Rita's advice. In March 2004 I call James's

ex-wife, Carol, a top medical practitioner. She and James have remained good friends after their split and I both like and admire her. She is calm and professional on the telephone. 'Don't worry, Nula. I'm sure it'll be fine. I'm going to arrange for him to see one of my colleagues.'

Only a few weeks later James and I are off to London to the Harley Street practice of the consultant Carol recommended.

We are shown into a beautiful Georgian room furnished with very fine antiques and I fill in a form the receptionist gives me, stating the details of James's health history. As we sit waiting to be called I think how odd it is that James still hasn't asked me why we're here or what we are doing. He has followed me, smiling, like a compliant child. It's as if we're on an outing and being at a doctor's office is nothing to do with him.

In spite of this I feel naively optimistic. Our visit, I think, will definitely sort out James's problem once and for all.

But the consultant's questions are bizarre.

'James, who is the Prime Minister and what is his name?'

'Do you know who the monarch of England is?'

'What is her name?'

'Who is the leader of the opposition party in the government?'

'Can you spell 'world' backwards?'

'Can you count back from twenty?'

'Do you know the capital of Germany?'

James just mumbles and stammers incomprehensibly. I increasingly dislike the consultant in his pinstripe suit and bow tie. I'm confused as to why he's asking such banal questions. Once he's finished he sits back in his chair and gives me a pompous and patronising look. When he speaks he doesn't think to include James, by so much as a glance in his direction.

'I think your husband has some form of dementia. I'm not quite sure what type. We'll need a scan and some tests before I'm positive.'

I can't speak for a minute. I feel as if he has hit me over the head with a cricket bat. Perhaps I've misunderstood him, not heard him properly.

'Pardon? What did you say?'

He was cool, matter-of-fact in his response. 'Yes, yes, I'm almost certain it's dementia.'

I can only repeat the word, seeking to understand what it is he's trying to tell me.

'It's a chronic disorder of the mental processes caused by a brain disease. Marked by disorders of personality and impaired reasoning.'

What is he talking about? Can't the man speak in plain English, and does he have to be so bloody cold in the way he says it? Anyway, I'm not taking anything in. My mind has frozen. I'm paralysed; shaking.

'There's no cure,' he adds.

He's speaking, moving his mouth, but I can't hear

anything, understand anything.

'I think we should get a second opinion. And I'll get you booked in for that. But I warn you, the prognosis is grim.' And then he twists the knife again. 'He may not have more than a year.'

'A year?'

'Yes, it's very similar to another case I had two years ago. A doctor living in the south of England. In fact, pretty much the same age as James. Presented much the same symptoms. He died within twelve months.'

My stomach tightens and I think I'm going to be sick. I've got to get out of this office.

The consultant stands up, now equally keen to be rid of us, it seems. At the door of his consulting room he doesn't offer a handshake or even a goodbye. James, though, smiles and thanks the man who has just given us the most dreadful news.

The receptionist, as cool and detached as her boss, asks for two hundred pounds.

'Would you like a receipt?' she asks.

I am in shock, and barely aware as we leave the Harley Street clinic that my darling James has just been given a death sentence. For me it is the introduction to a journey that will take me down a long road of sadistic hell that is the disease called dementia. Worse still, the person who was always there to share whatever life threw at me is unaware and no longer able to comfort or console me. It's a dreadful irony that the one person who was always my rock in times of difficulty was now not aware of the dreadful predicament I found myself in.

I didn't think that James had understood a word of what was said in the consulting room, but perhaps I am wrong. As we walk down the street he puts his arm around me – by now I'm in floods of tears – saying, 'Darling if I'm going to die you'll be okay. I've looked after you.'

Could it be that he understands that he's just been given a death sentence? And if so, how can he be taking it so calmly?

My heart is in shreds.

We walk on, until we coincidentally arrive at his favourite restaurant. Standing outside, James smiles and says, 'I'm hungry. I'd love something to eat, and a coffee.'

He never once refers to the consultant or asks me what the visit was about. I leave him tucking into his favourite Welsh rarebit and go to the cloakroom where the terror of it engulfs me. I collapse over the sink in tears. My reflection in the mirror looks back at me: white-faced with bloodshot, swollen eyes and blotchy skin. My head is reeling. I am so unprepared for this. I don't know how to deal with it. I'm terrified. What am I going to do?

I cannot begin to tell you how frightening the word dementia is, especially when you are not expecting to hear it. Rita had spoken of a possible tumour or a slight stroke, but she had not once mentioned dementia. Two hours ago

I walked into the Harley Street clinic thinking that I could be told that James had a brain lesion, or might have to have a course of chemotherapy at worst. But dementia? Isn't that what old people get? Not my James.

* * *

Carol arranges for a second opinion. I feel a glimmer of hope. Maybe the Harley Street quack has got it wrong. It could be a tumour after all, the lesser of two evils. A month later, at Addenbrooke's Hospital in Cambridge, after several tests and brain scans, the consultant, a professor of neurology, is – in contrast to the first consultant – warm and compassionate. Dressed in a T-shirt and jeans, he greets us with a handshake and jokes with James, smiling 'Hi James, this time I'm behind the camera and you're in front'. He chats and asks more questions, none of which James can answer. Having looked at all the results he hits us with the final blow.

'James, I'm afraid, has Pick's Disease. It's a very rare form of dementia that affects the frontal and temporal lobes of the brain. It affects less than 5 per cent of the population. Sufferers are often in the 45 to 60 age group, like James. He has all the characteristics: the slow deterioration of social skills, the changing personality, the impairment of his intellect, memory and language. You see, the cells are damaged in the frontal lobes which regulate our personalities, emotions and behaviour.'

The stark truth is that there is no cure. There are drugs, like Aricept, but they are really only of benefit in the very early stages and even then we are not certain they work. Sadly, he tells us that, shaking his head. James is too late for any drug treatment. The prognosis varies from patient to patient. 'They can live for anything between one and twelve years,' the consultant tells me gently.

'As James's dementia is Pick's, it will allow him to have a small window of awareness for a time. But it's a very, very small window.'

The doctor goes on to say that we still know very little about the disease. 'And even though we are researching all the time it's difficult, because we can only examine the brain fully after death.'

I want to keep him talking, to give me some hope, but he straightens up and says that's it. So no reasons, no cause, no surgery, no treatment, and – worst of all – no follow-up appointment. I'm on my own.

'There's nothing I, or anyone else, can do,' the man with compassionate eyes tells me. He finishes by saying, 'The disease is not kind, least of all, to the spouse. The only comforting thing I can give you is that, as far as we know, James won't be aware of it.'

I wail out loud. James continues to smile, even laugh, at the consultant as if he's being told some wonderful news.

Leaving, James reaches out and shakes the Prof's hand

as he leads us out into an empty grey corridor, a dead end with no route plan, no guide on how to navigate our way through the horrendous landmines of dementia country.

This was the beginning of our journey to hell.

8 : Sucking the Sweetness

But the tender grace of a day that is dead
Will never come back to me...
— Alfred Lord Tennyson

People react in different ways to a bleak diagnosis. Some respond with a busy flurry of research, a hope for a new miracle cure that never dies. Others decide to savour each moment they have left to them, sucking in the sweetness from each day. With Pick's Disease it was certain there really wasn't any hope at all for a cure, however hard I looked, and while James couldn't take the decision to suck the sweetness, I sure as hell was going to give him as much of it as I could.

With the official confirmation that James now has dementia and that there is no cure and no further treatment, I know there is nothing I nor anyone can do to bring my darling back to where he was before. We had shared a map of our past. The idea of losing him and navigating a future without him was beyond unbearable.

My witty, funny, brilliantly bright James, who has the most wonderful mind and most beautiful soul, is travelling at speed further and further away from me. How could I see him go through all this and not be able to explain to him or do anything to cure or comfort him? Our future was together. Both in our fifties, death was in the far, far distance, and anyway I always thought I would die long before him. Both my parents had died at 70. His parents lived into their late 80s.

That bastard dementia has gatecrashed our life and is taking away every wonderful thing we have. We had not asked for it and had done nothing to deserve it.

So why the fuck us?

Dementia, dementia. What is it? I still know very little. All I know is, it's a bloody cruel, sadistic disease, that has demolished my hopes, plans and dreams. It has taken away my life, twisted it and mangled it, and so it can claim another victim – two for the price of one.

As for James, dementia has launched a missile attack on his brain. First it robs him of his memory, then his ability to speak, then it progressively takes over his other functions, as it encroaches into the frontal lobes of his brain, leading him into the wilderness alone, until every last vestige of his dignity has disappeared.

So that's it. There's something so very final about dementia, so no wonder it has the stigma of taboo about it. Incurable, untreatable … so that even the consultant neurologist asks you not to bother to book in for another appointment. 'We've diagnosed you, now we're washing our hands of you. You're on your own now.' That is the message I'm getting.

After the shock wears off and the terrible truth begins to sink in over the next few days, I accept the situation with extreme reluctance. I have to refocus my thoughts and plans on the one positive glimmer I managed to glean from the consultant's talk: James would have a window – a limited one, it's true – but a window nonetheless. So I decide to fight the cruel dementia and to make the best of the time we have for James's sake – as well as my own – before the disease engulfs his mind completely.

I am going to go places with James, do things that he'll love, see the world, go to operas and concerts, spend this autumn of our time squeezing the last drop of togetherness and happiness from it. And we'll keep on doing it until the wretched disease beats us into submission.

* * *

I become, over the next five years, James's carer, nurse and mother. My role as wife and lover has to be surrendered, and is gone forever. Instead I become embroiled in a marathon battle with the bastard dementia, determined to hold onto every second of our life together. I include James in everything I do, for as long as possible, wanting to share and give him lovely, last experiences while he still has a window. So I carry on doing things normally, taking him to the cinema, the theatre, the opera and to concerts. I order his favourite food in restaurants and we drink the best wine.

Every day is precious, especially in the early stages. I bring him with me when I have to travel abroad for my work. I give huge tips to hotel porters to keep an eye on him and entertain him when I visit clients. They engage James in meaningless conversation and buy him a Guinness at the hotel bar, and when I return he greets me with outstretched arms and hugs me, with the biggest smile.

I take him to parties. On the dance-floor one time, a stranger who knows nothing about our situation, compliments us, saying, 'You make a handsome couple.' A gallon of sadness pours over me as she says it.

Every time we eat out in restaurants I look at James across the table with incredible nostalgia and remember past dinners when we had so much to talk about.

I'd brought him into my world of architects, design works and art; he'd shared his own world of film, drama and writing. We could never stop talking, talking, talking. So much love, so much sharing, so much laughter.

Now it is becoming impossible to communicate or engage in even the most basic conversation.

There are glimmers of the old James, and when they appear I greedily catch them up and hold them to my heart, even though it feels like this mixture of joy and nostalgia carries its own pain. We go to Paris, and while we're sitting in our favourite French restaurant he stuns me by speaking in fluent French to the waiter – James once more the debonair, clever, charming man he always was.

Then we're back to the mixture of words that make no sense, a new language that I'm trying to decipher, to glean whatever meaning I can so that I can understand his wants:

'Just to say to have really good on to keep – it would be great if we could get it – to say we have see here that's funny it bloody well different world – they don't know all of the – only me one and I got it – the other one it's only me but I haven't – I can't talk to anyone and that and that the best things to see if both of us to try the good things. No one tell you nothing to themselves on it. Remember me talking, talking nicely correctly comes in right. Two of them three of them, love it the wirld nobody, great guys – well it's good – later on first one to told me to see the whole things for it to see – you told me see I love it love it it's wirld held whole things – do again if you line [like] it's a good thing afterwards. Could up there – first certain wirlds be because I said I did but he's not there – two of them sitting on much as well welled – left it about it, all day day make sure of it – go up the wirlds – told him – all this was novel (awful) it be there…'.

* * *

Choosing the right fly has always been for James as satisfying and thrilling as the fishing itself. He relishes the process of finding exactly the best spot on the bank and selecting the best fly to lure the relevant fish, be it a wild salmon or a sea trout.

I take him to the wilds of Kerry to fly fish on Lough Currane. My brother Cyril, an award-winning fisherman who has even had a fly – the Murray Fly – named after him, has agreed to take James out on the lough.

It brings tears to my eyes as I watch the anticipation lighting James's face as he gets into the boat with his fishing gear. It is worth everything to give him that joy. But later, sitting in the middle of the lough, I notice immediately that his fingers are clumsy and he cannot coordinate the tying of his fly onto the line. I can't help remembering how, in past years, he tied his fly in seconds and cast. It was poetry in motion to watch him swishing out his line over a lake or a river in his beautiful balletic way, to allow his fly to fall gently – barely touching the water – and causing hardly a ripple on the surface.

I'm taken back to the day, years before, when he caught a ten-pound wild salmon, and the complete delight on James's face when he held it up. How we laughed later when he told his friends over dinner about his catch – and how the salmon grew heavier in weight with each telling.

Now my brother has to do it all – tie the fly and help James cast. Another reminder of how much dementia has taken away.

* * *

James has always been coolly romantic. He'd make love to me before taking me out to dinner, then buy the best bottle of wine to have with it, to celebrate our good luck in having each other. At other times he'd come home bearing a recently published book or buy a little sketch drawing or painting he thought I might like.

He would always point out something beautiful in nature – a snowdrop fighting its way through the frozen ground to bloom in the freezing temperatures or wondering just how it was that an acorn could become a huge tree.

He knew I didn't like cultivated, shop-bought flowers, so used to go to great efforts to get the florist to send me wild flowers on my birthday. Often, too, while walking the dogs he would pick little bunches of cornflowers or cowslips and cuttings from trees and give them to me on his return.

Oddly perhaps, considering his love of plants, James has never been much of a gardener. When he plants sweet pea seeds I don't take a whole lot of notice, little realising that they'll germinate and grow over six feet tall over the next months, their fragile foliage intertwined around a high trellis. James becomes obsessive about watering them daily and pruning the dead flowers.

I'm stunned when these sweet peas produce an abundance of beautifully scented flowers in hues of white, pink, red and purple. When I return home in the evening I find sweet peas all over the house: in vases, cups, mugs, jugs, sitting on window ledges, tables, and in my study. The delicate scent of them wafts throughout.

Most precious of all, but also most heartbreaking, is when I leave for work in the mornings and find little bouquets of sweet peas on the seat and dashboard of my car.

It is his only way of telling me he loves me.

9 : Getting Harder

So if, my dear, there sometimes seem to be
Old bridges breaking between you and me

Never fear. We may let the scaffolds fall
Confident that we have built our wall.
                              – Seamus Heaney

When it becomes too difficult living in our isolated country house, James and I move into a flat in the centre of Dublin. My office is around the corner, so it makes looking after James much easier: this way I can pop home to check on him at lunchtimes. I hope that having city life around him will keep him stimulated, and I often bring him into the office with me for a coffee, if I have a quiet moment, to make him feel included.

In the early days after diagnosis, his dropping by for coffee doesn't disrupt the office. Anna, our 25-year-old receptionist, fusses over him, making sure to offer him his favourite biscuits. But then the visits escalate and very soon he starts to call in at odd times, not all of which are convenient. Anna is very good at persuading him to return home when this is the case.

Then the sandwiches begin to arrive. In the past, James would always make one for my lunch on the days when we were both working from home, but now he brings them to the office at peculiar times, sometimes in the early morning or late afternoon, or evenings when I am working late. At first they're ham, cheese and tomato, the bread cut to uneven degrees of thickness, the butter revoltingly applied in thick lumps and seeping out of the sides of the sandwich.

Then the sandwiches become weirder. James arrives with Mouse, our Jack Russell, laughing in his dementia way, bearing bread covered in jam, mayonnaise, mustard and whatever else he can find in the kitchen cupboard.

I realise we made the mistake, when James first started bringing them in, of accepting the sandwiches. But I always feel heartbroken that he is trying to have my company, and thinks he is helping by making sure I have something to eat.

At some point I realise that I have to take on more professional help. I've been relying so far on my cleaner, Irina, who has filled in here and there with James on the few occasions I dare go away for work. She works enormously hard, and has been the most amazing support to me, but now – due to James's sudden and bizarre reaction to her – I will have to find other help.

Irina is a twenty-eight-year-old Lithuanian with peroxide blonde hair showing two inches of dark roots, and indecently short skirts. She is also the kindest, hardest worker you can imagine who has raised three kids and learned to speak English more than competently after arriving in Ireland as a penniless, illiterate and pregnant immigrant several years ago.

On one particular day that will forever stay in my mind, Irina comes by to collect £500 in cash, which includes her Christmas bonus. I offer her a Christmas drink and pass her a bottle of vodka from the cupboard. Soon she is sharing her family troubles with me, sitting at the kitchen table while I sort out my clothes for our trip to Florida. Suddenly I realise she has drunk most of the bottle. Worried, I immediately suggest Irina gets herself home, insisting, looking at the state of her, that she takes a taxi.

I ask James to escort her for the five-minute walk to the taxi rank and he willingly obliges, putting on his dark-grey coat and winding his scarf around his neck, and they set out. What happens after that is a story worthy of a Carry On film. The old James would have laughed till his sides ached but this new James is not amused.

It seems that Irina and James, walking along the road to the taxi rank, were spotted by two policemen on patrol. What is a relatively posh street by day becomes a haunt for prostitutes at night, and it isn't hard to see that the peroxide blonde Irina, and the conservatively respectable James, must have seemed like a classic hooker with her client.

One of the policemen asks James his name. James is silent. Irina, in her inebriated state, tells the cop to 'piss off'. They are bundled into a squad car and driven to the police station, Irina charged with being abusive, James with 'using the services of a prostitute in a public area and refusing to give his name'. It doesn't help their case that £500 in cash is found on Irina.

It doesn't take long, though, before the policeman examining James realises that something isn't quite right about him and eventually finds a card in his coat with my details on it. He calls me, the matter is quickly cleared up, and James is brought back home by two mortified and apologetic policemen.

If we could only have laughed things off as we would have done in the old days! Instead, James becomes very aggressive towards Irina and refuses to allow her ever to enter the flat again.

After that, James refuses to accept help from agency carers, accusing them of stealing from him and, once, even threatening to hit one of them.

* * *

All the while trying to work and run a business, with James rapidly deteriorating, is turning into a nightmare. The situation is worsening and dementia is taking over both our lives.

When I offer to take on a project on the other side of Ireland it becomes the last straw. I leave James with a friend in the morning, arranging to pick him up later in the day.

But when I get to the site, having driven the four hours to it, the clients tell me they have a family emergency and need to reschedule their appointment for the next morning. I arrange to stay at a friend's cottage but know that I can't possibly leave James for the night, so I drive the four hours back to Dublin, pick him up with his belongings, and drive across the country once more to the cottage. I have no time to cook a proper meal so bring a sandwich for James to eat in the car while I drive.

James looks at the sandwich, turns it over, inspects the contents and then refuses to eat it. He starts to shout at me, 'This is shit, shit, shit!' then he throws the sandwich onto the floor of the car and stamps his foot on it.

Stressed out and furious, I lose it. I pull over to the side of the road, stop the car, and yell at him, 'For fuck's sake, why did you do that? It's a perfectly good free range chicken sandwich!' I grab him by the arm. 'Do you realise I've driven twelve hours today just to have you with me and to make sure you're safe?' He meets my stare blankly. 'I'm working flat out to keep us both. I have a job to do and your moaning about a sandwich is not helping!'

The petulant, overtired child that was James a moment ago is now looking confused. He has no idea what I'm talking about or why I'm shouting at him. I put my head on the steering wheel and sob with frustration.

Later, when we arrive at the cottage, James becomes disorientated and starts to pace the room. I try to reassure him that it's only for one night but he doesn't understand. I put him to bed and get in beside him, but even sleep is impossible as James gets up several times in the night and tries to get outside.

In the morning I shower him, dress him and give him his breakfast before leaving him with a friend, while I try my best to sound on top of things at my client meeting. Every bit of my body and brain is shattered. I feel I'm being pushed inexorably over the edge.

Later my friend telephones me, concerned. 'You left the gas on and your overnight bag behind. Nula, I'm worried about you. You can't go on like this. I've just had him for half a day and I'm exhausted. What must it be like for you? He's too much for you to manage on your own while you're trying to work as well, you must see that. It's going to kill you!'

I know she's right, but I am not giving up on James. And I can't give up earning either so I'll just have to do the best I can.

The trouble is that even relaxation times aren't relaxing. There is no respite after a long day's work. When all I want to do is curl up in front of the television, James makes it impossible. There's no way I can watch a film from beginning to end as he interrupts constantly with his ceaseless, meaningless chatter. My frustration at not being able to make sense of it grows daily. I search for meaning and sometimes pick up a thread here and there, a clue as to

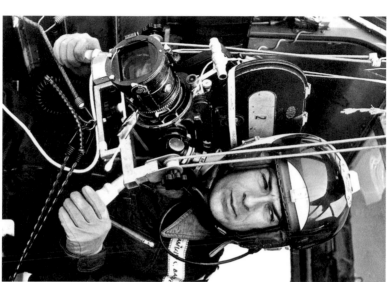

James filming for BBC *Panorama* in post-war Vietnam, 1987

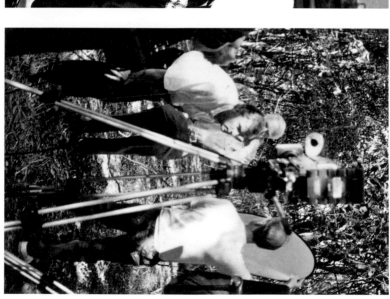

James directing 'Early Man' in Kenya, Walter Cronkite alongside him, 1992

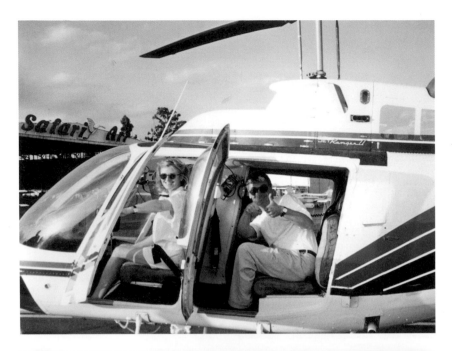

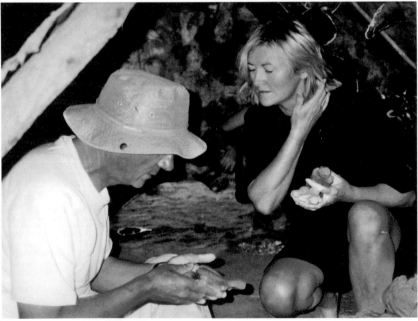

Top. James impressing me with a helicopter ride over Meru and Mwingi National Reserves, Kenya, 1992
Bottom: James directing me on the set of *Early Man* in Kenya, 1992

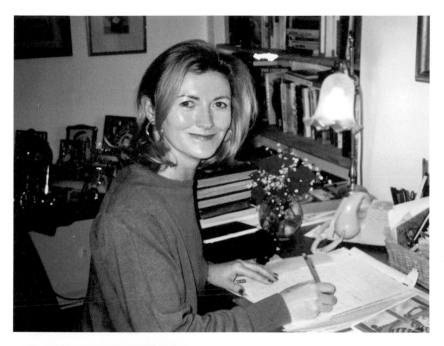

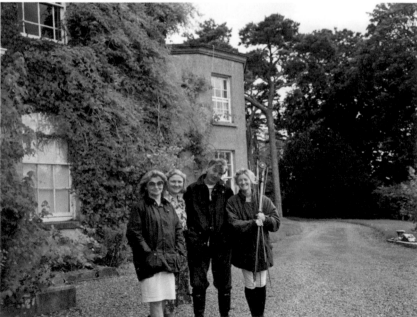

Top. Catching up with paperwork at home in Ireland, 1993
Bottom: Just back from fishing to a surprise visit from my mother and sister
Stasia, 1994

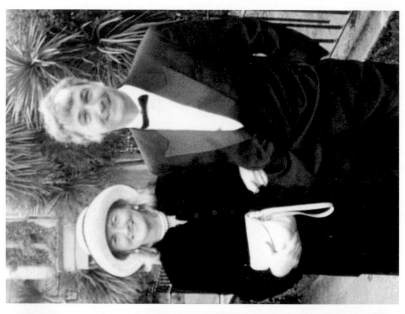

All dressed up for a friend's wedding, 1998

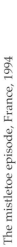

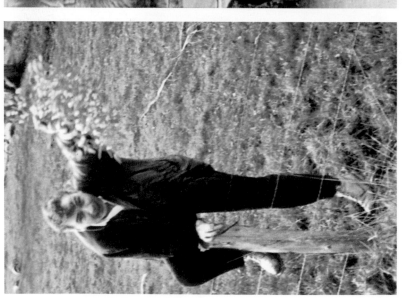

The mistletoe episode, France, 1994

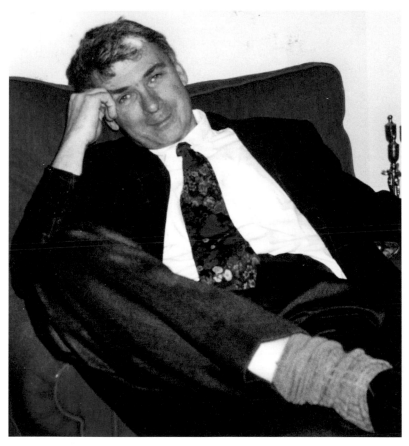

Relaxing after a friend's birthday party, Connemara, 1998

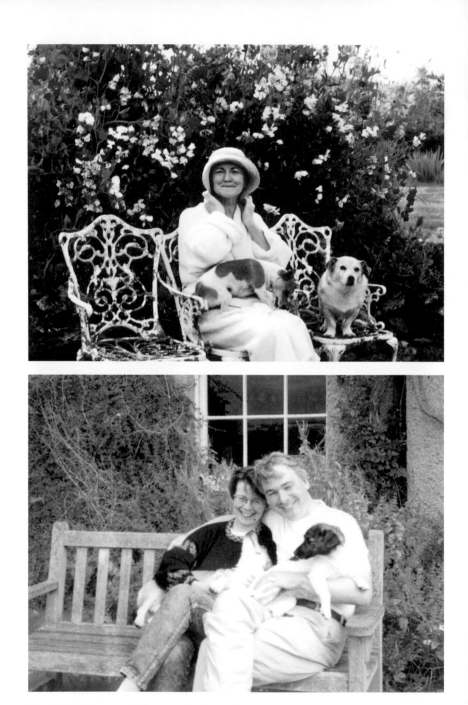

Top. With Mouse and Spanny in front of James's sweetpeas
Bottom: James with cousin Marion and my adored Lucy

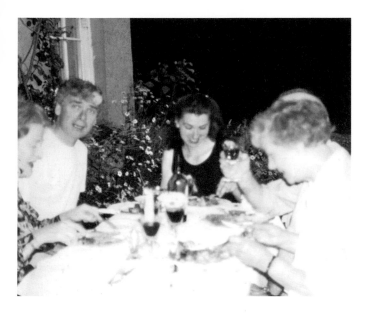

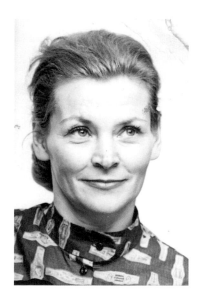

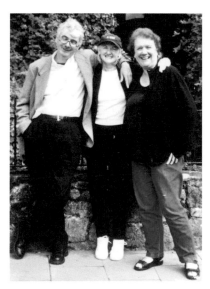

Top. James with his mother Bridget celebrating his sister Maureen's graduation
Bottom. Nula's mother Maura in her sixties; James and Nula with James's sister Margaret

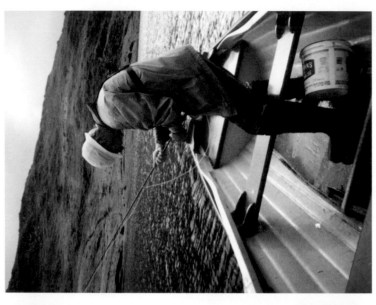

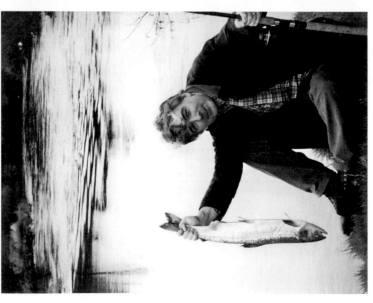

Two fishing trips. Left, James proudly displaying his wild salmon catch, in 2000. And right, on his last fishing trip in 2009 five years after his diagnosis what he is trying to convey.

'Just to say to have a really good on to keep it would be great if we could get it. To say have see here that's funny it bloody well different world they don't know all of them only me, one and only it got the other one, it's only me but I haven't. I can't talk to anyone and that and that the best things to see it both of us both to try it the good things. No one tells me nothing to themselves on it. Two of them three them love it the world. It's a good thing afterwards nobody obviously you are seed, hold it load of your out to see how long when it comes lovely things. Love beautiful things up there afterwards just us no one I wirld gets us nobody, nobody says well it's great … say to just … it's great to see it, say to, it's be great it's a lovely great things you told me you know it, we're here this think thing, load of little shits, nobody can do, very nicely see it it comes two of it , you'll see beautiful things up their in wirld mini mini La Boheme, that would be great. I'm thinking me you how won't see wirld and be another this place kleeps [keeps], good thing for it, me to you, me me to you you to me it would be great'

It tears me apart watching him trying to communicate with me. I can get the gist sometimes of what he's trying to say: 'We have each other and we love each other. We don't need any other person. No one else understands.'

There's a glimmer of understanding there, I'm sure of it. He is trying to tell me he knows but dementia is putting him in a horrible place with the wrong mind.

10 : Travels and the Difficulties of Out and About

When you reach the end of your rope, tie a knot in it and hang on
– Franklin D. Roosevelt

I would love to take James skiing. It was a much loved annual hobby before I met him. He would go away with television friends post-Christmas, the quietest time in the media world, for several weeks and ski off piste. But because of my work commitments I can't take the time off, and I can't let him go on his own.

Instead I take him on a fishing trip to Mayo's Lough Arrow for the mayfly season. Here trout go into a frenzied feeding session that ensures great fishing. It makes it easy for even the poorest fisherman to catch a fish. I know it will be my final opportunity to give him that one last pleasure, without anyone else needing to be with us.

From years of accompanying him on previous fishing trips I have become adept at tying flies. We are ready to set out on a boat with rods at the ready when suddenly James lurches to the side clutching his stomach in obvious pain. With no toilet facilities nearby he leans over a nearby bench.

Within seconds he's overwhelmed with a horrible bout of diarrhoea. Visibly upset he returns to the car and refuses to let me help him. I have no choice but to drive the three hours back to Dublin with the stench of diarrhoea overpowering the pair of us.

* * *

I'm doing my best to travel with James to familiar places where he can feel relaxed and at ease. However it is getting increasingly difficult. Airport security is a nightmare, especially after 9/11.

'Sir, could you remove your jacket and your shoes?'

James refuses.

The man with a gun at his side repeats the question. James responds with, 'Fuck, fuck, fuck.'

He laughs inappropriately and now the man starts to get impatient. I sense this could result in James being arrested.

I plead with the official, 'Please, please understand, my husband's got dementia!'

But the man, whose impression is no doubt that the handsome refusenik is most likely a terrorist, finds it hard to understand that this youngish, handsome, normal-looking individual could possibly have dementia.

After this one particularly stressful occasion I always travel with a doctor's note stating that James has Pick's Disease.

And it's not just public transport that's a problem. I'm finding that driving with James is becoming extremely difficult, even dangerous. As cars approach, passing on the other side of the road, he raises his arms in fear, thinking they're going to crash into us. No matter how slowly I drive or how much I try to reassure him, he still panics. I'm starting to fear I'll end up crashing the car and killing someone.

I'm losing my sense of humour and James is losing all inhibition. That filter in his mind has ceased to work.

If we're out shopping or in a public place he'll call out insulting things to passers-by. If a girl walks past with a trendy rip in her jeans, he'll say to her, pointing: 'You can't wear those!' Even worse is when a large man passes and he bellows: 'You're too fat!' It is impossible to steer him away or avoid pitfalls, as there is rarely a pattern or logic to his pointing things out. He randomly laughs at nothing and he no longer laughs when something is genuinely amusing. He picks up items in a shop and puts them in his pocket.

No less embarrassing and even more stressful are those incidents when James becomes aggressive. He regularly tells people to 'fuck off', and will almost always cross the road without checking if it's safe. I lurch forward in horror when a car only just stops in time, screeching to a halt as James wanders out in front of it. James lashes out in fury, thumping the bonnet and enraging the driver, swearing at the man as if only he, James, has right of way across the busy road.

The other time he becomes obstreperous is when he has to wear an incontinence pad on long journeys. After the mayfly fishing trip I insist on him wearing his pads. But it's a constant battle. After I finally manage to persuade him he needs to wear one, he is perfectly liable to remove the soiled pad in a public place and fling it, shouting, 'fuck shit!', to the horror of onlookers. Just as bad are the times when he needs to go, and because there is that lack of filter – which would moderate normal people's behaviour – he just takes down his trousers and pees where he stands.

To prevent this, I first have to plan our every move, trying before anything else to find a toilet, then I have to ask a man, a stranger, to take him in. Most of the time James forgets I'm outside waiting for him and I have to call out, 'James, I'm here.' Then he will invariably ignore me and I have to ask a stranger to go in and tell my husband I'm outside. 'He's got dementia,' I explain. There are times I have to go in myself, braving strange looks from men at the urinals.

Restaurants have ceased being anything but stressful. The evening in Paris where James spoke French in such a debonair way to the waiter seems part of another era now.

When the waiter reads out the specials James says, 'yes' to all of them. I order what I think he'll like but if it's not what he's expecting when it arrives, he shoves the plate to the edge of the table and says, 'fuck fuck.'

The real sadness, and the start of our growing isolation,

is when even entertaining at home becomes too stressful to be worth it. James is at first able to enjoy the company of a small group of our close friends around the table, joining in the conversation with his senseless chat for a short while.

But as the meal progresses it becomes clear that his language skills are now so impaired and his words so mangled that it is difficult and exhausting to include him. Our guests carry on chatting regardless until, at some point, James, feeling frustrated, annoyed and uninhibited, stands up and leaves the table. He paces the floor for a time and keeps looking at his watch, no matter how early it is, before returning to the table, where he stands over our guests and says angrily, 'It's time you fuckers left.'

Our friends try to placate him, but all their efforts at humouring him – 'Ah, James, please, please stay with us' – are in vain. He continues pacing the floor, looking angry and frustrated, until finally they leave, not wanting to stress him further. They understand what is going on and laugh away my embarrassment.

Finally I have to stop inviting friends to our home. Alone with James, I continue to try to communicate with him, responding to his endless chatter and forever trying to make sense of it. It is exhausting, especially after a long working day, but I never give up – desperate to hold onto any little bit of him.

* * *

Music is one of the last things I won't give up on for James. In the early stages of dementia he would weep copiously every time I played an opera CD, *Tosca, La Bohème* especially, and he still responds viscerally to what has always been one of the greatest joys in his life.

Sometimes he annoys opera-goers by getting up and walking out in the middle of an aria, and in Verona he blocked the view of the audience seated behind us by wearing his straw hat throughout the performance, which he refused to take off. Some see the funny side and glance at each other, smiling; others get cross and huff a little.

Glyndebourne is a nightmare. I realise almost as soon as we arrive that I never should have booked it. There is something so richly formal and glamorous about the occasion, everyone dressed in their best clothes: men in black tie, women sparkling with jewels, and too great a risk of James misbehaving, something the poor lamb would be almost certain to do. I had thought it all through beforehand and reasoned that it would probably be more problematic if we were to sit with picnickers in the gardens as James would show little inhibition if he needed the toilet and might well drop his trousers there and then. I couldn't risk that so I'd booked a table in the dining hall.

Oh dear. Everyone is looking at us askance and their glances aren't forgiving or benign – or at least I don't read them that way in my embarrassed state. James, presented with the food I have ordered for him has just shouted, 'Fuck, this is shit, shit, shit, fuck!'

I try to placate him, feeling every flinty eye in the room upon us, but it only makes him more angry and he repeats his tirade in his loudest voice: 'Shit, shit! Fuck!'

I cringe with embarrassment, feeling the disdain of everyone in the hall, then suddenly I think, 'Fuck them. All that matters is that James is getting some enjoyment from the day.'

Things are a whole different ballgame when we go to a Leonard Cohen concert together. There is nothing stiff and formal about the event so we both feel more carefree.

In the early stages of his dementia James persistently used to sing the opening lines of 'I Can't Forget': 'I stumbled out of bed / I got ready for the struggle / I smoked a cigarette / And I tightened up my gut,' and he would laugh. He had a special love and respect for Cohen, a poet, marvelling at how he could spend a whole year composing one song, just to get it absolutely right.

This time my planning works a treat. I have hired a wheelchair for the occasion and now I wheel James through the throng of concertgoers and he's smiling and enjoying it, as if he understands that it'll be our best way to get close to the front of the stage.

Later, I forget to put the break on when I go to the bar to get us a glass of wine but an experienced wheelchair user recognises my mistake and rushes to help. James beams up at him, laughing like I haven't seen him laugh for ages and chats in his nonsensical language. Everyone is laughing, everyone is happy, and my heart sings to be there in the company of supportive strangers.

We continue to visit as many places as we can, so keen am I to fill enough of James's bucket list as possible before the window closes. We fly to Prague to hear Verdi's *Nabucco*. James gets up in the middle of an aria to go to the toilet and annoys the people sitting behind us. On the Charles Bridge a cartoonist draws his portrait. Sadly he has no recollection of our previous visits, researching Mozart.

In Paris we go to an auction room. In the past James loved browsing around auction rooms hoping to spot something interesting. A painting catches James's eye, of three down-at-heel musicians playing violins outside a wealthy home. He loves it and I bid for it. It costs me more than I can really afford, but he loves it and that's all that matters.

11 : Isolation

And it's partner found, it's partner lost
And it's hell to pay when the fiddler stops
— Leonard Cohen

Dementia is destroying everything. My marriage, my dreams, my finances, even myself. Everything is subsumed by the soul-crushing grind of being a carer to the empty shell that is now my darling James.

There's very little conversation any more. The daily boredom of trying to find things that will give him pleasure closes in. I put on his much loved operas. The one he loves most is *La Bohème*. He watches it over and over again and sobs.

He's now calling Mouse, our little Jack Russell, Minnie, which is his version of Mimi, and talks to her non-stop in his own language:

'Minnie La Boheme you me means as well that far to very good nicely good things afterwards whole things – years years as well away so many things in the wirld I was things in the wirld ....'

Walking to the park with Mouse. Feeding the ducks. The simple pleasure of taking him for a coffee to a nearby café turns out to be stressful. He knocks over his cup, spills coffee all over his trousers and top. I apologise. The Polish waiter knows us by now and rushes to help. He says, 'It doesn't matter'. He brings more coffee. James chats to the waiter. Neither understand the other. I smile to myself. James would have seen the funny side.

We return home. I undress James, take off the soiled shirt and trousers. And another battle resumes to allow me to shower him and put on clean clothes. I'm exhausted and emotionally drained. Sitting on the edge of the bed I break down and cry. I've just remembered it's my birthday.

Only too soon we cease to go out very much at all. It's not worth the stress and it's obvious James is getting little or no pleasure any more.

My work suffers as I can't always take James with me, nor can I leave him for any great length of time. Working abroad or having to travel any distance at all becomes impossible, so increasingly I turn down projects. Inevitably offers of work begin to dwindle.

James's language, what's left of it, is becoming more aggressive.

'First up there – fucking shit certain wirlds sitting on much as well – left it about sitting there – to too all day day make sure if it go up the way – bastard I sed told him all this was bloody things all money – liked it – tell of it ...'

In outside company there is an embarrassment around his illness and I hate the social and intellectual humiliation of my once brilliant husband being ostracised in conversation. As his window closes down I don't want the world to see him this way, so to protect him I stop going out. We become ever more isolated, struggling along in our leaking ship as the months pass.

I have to keep an ever-closer eye on James. He's taken to going through all our personal papers, something he'd never have done in the past. One day I come home to find that all my papers, along with my diary and passport, have disappeared. He's thrown away a lot of his own scripts and documents too. I can't find any of it.

I'm hardly getting any sleep. How I'm functioning at all is a miracle. James might get out of bed at 3am to make toast or he'll appear at my bedside in the middle of the night with a breakfast tray of inedible food. Soon I learn to turn off the electricity at night and hide all the appliances.

He's now taken to waking up in the night and getting fully dressed, then coming back to bed. I'm too exhausted to coax him to remove his clothes and put his pyjamas on. It's easier to leave him. What a sight we look. James in bed fully dressed in a jacket, shirt and tie, me in a nightie!

I laugh.

It's that or cry!

He carries a leather bag everywhere. It's full of old papers that, he thinks, are important to him. One such article is a review of a documentary, The Kuru Mystery, he made over twenty-five years ago. He tells me and the postman he filmed it last week.

My friend Colette invites us both over to her flat for James's birthday dinner. She makes a comment, 'Do you realise there are three of you in this marriage, you, James and dementia? No wonder you're mentally worn down and exhausted.'

Maureen, James's sister, telephones me, 'I'm coming over for the weekend to give you a break'.

She arrives full of enthusiasm to share a few days with James. On the first day of her stay, he yells at her, 'Get the hell out of here!'. It's heartbreaking knowing how much he loved her, and how he was so proud of her when she graduated with a first class honours law degree. Now all forgotten in the haze of dementia.

It has become routine to wake up in the early hours to find the bed soaked in urine. I try to wake James, gently coaxing him from his deep sleep. When I do, he becomes really angry and confused, refusing to move, content to lie in a urine-soaked bed. I persist, pleading with him, 'Darling, the bed is soaking wet. I must change the sheets.' He lashes out at me, 'Fuck, fuck! No, no, no.' It's a battle to get his wet pyjamas off. Then, as soon as I've washed him and changed the bed linen I have another battle to persuade him to use the toilet and put on an incontinence pad. Finally, we're back in bed; I'm exhausted and it's nearly morning, and another day needs to be got through.

Forget about having any intimate life at all. I'm too

exhausted to even contemplate such a thing. Sometimes James reaches over to me in an attempt to make love but then he forgets why he's done so. I just lie there and replay all the good times we've had. Sometimes I feel guilty that I haven't tried to give him this one last pleasure. It's impossible, though. The old, passionate me has lost all desire – all the beauty of our love snuffed out, eaten up by the bastard dementia.

If I try to cut his hair or insist on giving him a bath he fights me all the way. He's six feet tall and the smallest task becomes a logistical nightmare. It is like dealing with a small petulant toddler when I have to shower him, change his clothes or cut his nails, although it's so much worse as this child is huge and much harder to handle.

I use every kind of gentle persuasion to get him to allow me to undress him after he's been incontinent. Finally, both of us naked, we stand together in the shower and I wash his hair and body. Sometimes I laugh out loud to see the pair of us reflected in the bathroom mirror. There's something almost comically ironic to remember how, in the past, a similar scene would have been such a romantically intimate experience.

12 : The Care Home Beckons

The breath of night like death did flow – Percy Shelley

Finally social workers and our doctor intervene: 'James needs full-time care provided by professional carers. You cannot manage him any more.'

The doctor – taking in the sight of me – warns that carers often die before their patients. I'm shocked that he's noticed such a change in me. Driven to the brink of collapse by sleepless nights and the daily stress of dealing with James over the past five years – not to mention my work – has caused me to lose over a stone in weight.

Dementia has taken over everything. Our finances, our dreams, our marriage and my sense of self. Now they are telling me I can no longer cope alone. The only solution is for James to be put into full-time care.

Immediately I know this is the cruellest, toughest decision I have ever had to take in my life.

I feel I have failed. I feel utterly defeated.

I am given a list of care homes.

Visiting them turns out to be far more horrific than I could ever have imagined. The first home is shocking. The sight of old people huddled in sodden chairs, looking into space while a television in the corner blares and flickers unwatched, is pitiful. I find out that the harassed, low paid carers are only allotted fifteen minutes per patient.

The second home is no better. As I walk into the entrance hall the smell of urine and boiled cabbage hits me so violently I can hardly breathe. My dog Mouse's boarding kennels are a luxury hotel compared to this.

Depressed, I return home.

Finally, my sister-in-law Maureen suggests a care home in England that specialises solely in dementia. She has heard good things about it.

As soon as I enter the home I know that this is probably the best there is. The entrance is like walking into a welcoming family hallway. It is small and intimate, and smells clean.

Sara, the nursing manager, shows me round. There is a buzz of activity with music playing, and entertainment and art classes are going on. There are cats and dogs wandering around, giving the place a homely feel. She points out the picture boards outside each patient's room. 'Here we show patients' past life, their occupation, their families, music they enjoyed and their hobbies, with photographs to remind them of who they were. It helps to give us, the carers – as well as the visitors – an indication of a patient's personality.'

This is a huge comfort to me. Any place that respects the patients, remembering that they are real people with a past life – a life outside dementia – is one I think I might be able to live with.

But still I waver.

Sara, sensing my reluctance to make a decision, sits me down and runs through each of the positives with me. 'I assure you it will be the best for James. We have enough staff to care for him twenty-four hours a day, who never get tired, never lose their patience. They can return home, have another life, get a good night's sleep and return here refreshed the next day. You cannot do this.'

She adds, 'And most importantly we can get to know the real James before dementia completely claims him.'

Her last sentence convinces me, and I admit I'm beaten. I sign on the dotted line and return home with a heavy heart.

When I'm back home in Ireland I go on to autopilot, mechanically sorting through things, ordering name tapes and sewing them on James's clothes, giving the ones he's not taking to a charity shop. My friend comments, 'The tramps in Dublin will be very stylish walking around in James's Italian jackets.'

I am awash with sadness. I pack his case and fold each piece of clothing, remembering how I used to do it in the past before he went away to film. This time there's no film, and no coming back.

We spend two nights in a country house hotel we used to love, at the edge of the ocean. We walk the sandy beach.

We come across a dead gull entangled in fishing tackle. I see it as a mirror of our life. We too are trapped – in a mesh of dementia.

We go for a walk in the nearby woods, the smell of autumn pervades. I fill our pockets with chestnuts, just as James would do in the earlier stages of his illness when he was out walking the dogs. He revelled in the fat, shiny fullness of the autumn fruit and offered them to strangers he met as if they were precious gifts.

We have our last dinner together. I order his favourite food and the best wine. I'm suffocating in sadness.

Worried that James might be incontinent I put plastic over the bottom sheet. In bed I tuck my knees under him, 'spoons' we called it in the past, and wrap my arms around him. James, now lost in dementia, is unresponsive and pushes me away.

13 : Listing the Last Times

Love won't be tampered with, love won't go away.
Push it to one side and it creeps to the other…
— *Isak Dinesen*

N o-one says goodbye to James when we leave Ireland. I don't think my family know what to do or say. It is as if he's become a non-person. If he had been diagnosed with cancer they would see him as a brave battler, but dementia frightens them. It would have been an unsettling farewell in any case; with everyone feeling upset at the knowledge that this is James's final journey, and he's never coming back.

My friend Colette is with me, though; I can't do this alone. As we stand waiting for the hydrofoil, James doesn't once ask me where we are going or why we are making the crossing. As I look back I think about how excited he and I were coming to Dublin just a few years before. So full of hope, fizzing with plans and ideas. He'd been commissioned by the Irish Film Board to write a screenplay for a documentary drama that he would go on to direct. Now all I can think about is how this is the last time he'll see his home country; the last time he'll go on a boat; the last time he'll travel through England in a car. With every minute, it feels there is another 'last time' added to the list.

Guilt dogs my footsteps. James follows me onto the boat, smiling and trusting like a child, happy to travel anywhere as long as he is with me. There have been many times over the past few years when I've felt my heart breaking, but this is one of the worst. I feel like a traitor. It really does seem that James, so sweet and compliant, is following me like a lamb to the slaughter.

Once on board Colette says, 'I'm going to get James a Guinness.'

He's grown rather fond of the drink and I give him a glass each evening to help him settle. She adds a small whiskey to the pint and he drinks it with a smile, laughing and talking in his nonsensical language. He thinks that we are out for a social drink. I smile back at him and my stomach churns.

We are in the car on the way to the care home in Hertfordshire. I am stunned to hear James read out the motorway signs – Birmingham; Watford; London – and he claps his hands with joy, shouting 'lovely, lovely' as we draw closer to London, a city he loves.

I think back to the professor who diagnosed him just five agonisingly short years ago, explaining how there would be a 'window' that would never entirely close. I have felt the aperture narrowing with every month of James's decline into dementia, but there are times like this when I get a glimmer of cognition. It is understandable that he should react to the words and the names – after all, he's lived and filmed in London and other major cities in the UK for most of his working life.

Much of the drive passes in silence. To lighten the mood, Colette puts on a selection of James's favourite music and sings along to J.J. Cale's 'Wish I had not said that': 'You don't come here too often / You make my day when you come around / You know I love you something awful / You're a diamond I have found.' I remember how we danced to this song at a friend's summer garden party soon after we met, and the intense thrill and passion I felt. I knew in that moment I'd found the love of my life. After a challenging background, to find this love was beyond amazing.

We stop several times to allow James to use the toilet. At one service station he refuses to wear his incontinence pad and throws it away. After that we are faced with the nightmare of stopping in a lay-by in torrential rain. Once James is outside the car, the traffic roaring past terrifies him so much he refuses to go. We stand on the verge for what seems like ages, soaked to the skin. We must make a strange sight – me holding his penis, reassuring him that it's okay – so much so that a couple of drivers hoot their horns aggressively as they pass.

* * *

Sara, the manager of the care home, puts an arm around James's shoulder. 'How lovely to see you, James. Welcome!' She gives him a huge smile. 'You're going to stay with us for a while.' He smiles back at her.

I made a huge effort on my previous visit to make his room feel familiar and comfortable, making sure he had his favourite chair, a small side table and various mementos. I had photographs enlarged of his and our past life and had covered the walls with them, hoping that they would give him some reminder of who he was. On top of his chest of drawers I put his radio and cassette player with his favourite CDs, and his television is on the wall opposite his chair. On the wall facing his bed, I hung the painting he adores – the one we bought at the Paris auction – of three musicians, knowing it will be the first thing he'll see each morning and the last at night.

He stands looking around the room, confused and bewildered.

Tea and cake is brought in on a tray, and while we eat and drink I don't take my eyes off James. I am watching for any reaction that might signal he is aware of our plan. But there is nothing – no sign at all that he knows this is his new home or that he'll be here for ever.

A little later, Sara draws me aside and whispers, 'When you leave, don't say goodbye. Just walk away. It'll be less confusing for him.'

This sends me into a panic. How can I not say goodbye?

In my agitation I do everything possible to delay my departure, moving around the room nervously, fiddling with things. I rearrange his clothes in the wardrobe; refold his underwear in his chest of drawers; arrange his photograph books and place them near his armchair; open a box of chocolates and put them on his side table.

I put on *The Marriage of Figaro*. On hearing his favourite Mozart opera, James gets up from his chair and stands in the middle of the room. Without the slightest inhibition he begins to conduct the music, a huge smile on his face as he looks at me and Colette. I can't breathe. I move to wrap my arms around his body and hold him tight so he can't see me cry.

I want to run out of the room with him and take him far away from the world of care homes and dementia.

Colette gently peels him from me, putting her arms around me and leading me out of his room. I look back to see James still conducting, oblivious to my leaving. Outside I break down completely. This is it. I have betrayed James by handing him over to strangers. This is the end. I know I will never share a home or a life with him again. The thought sends me into a spiral of hysterical sobbing. 'I can't do this. I can't do this. This is not right.'

Now Colette sits me in the car. She firmly reassures me, 'Nulsie, this is the best place for him. You cannot manage him anymore. It's not fair on James. You've not been able to care for him properly for a long time. He needs professional

care. Let's just try it for a couple of weeks. It will give you
some respite. You're exhausted. Look at you. You look like
a cadaver with all the weight you've lost. Caring for James
has taken a huge toll on your health. It's you I'm worried
about, not James, he will be fine. He will be well taken care
of.'

She talked on, 'This is the best for both of you. He will
have his own space and lots of carers who have the time,
patience and stamina to chat and look after him, and more
importantly, it will give you time to recover and get your
health back.'

It was no good – I didn't want to hear. The life we had
together had been cruelly taken away.

14 : Grief and Letting Go

We are hence, we are gone, as though we had not been there.
– Algernon Swinburne

The knowledge that we will never live together again annihilates me. I feel devastated over the next days and weeks. No-one can convince me that this is for the best, not even James's 84-year-old mother Brigid calling every day to tell me: 'Darling, you've done the right thing by him. He's safe and cared for. Don't keep beating yourself up like this.' But I do.

I wallow in 'no mores':

No more James and Nula.

No more living together.

No more hugging each other to sleep.

No more smiling face coming through my door.

No more arms outstretched to greet me.

No more hearing that beautiful voice call out to me.

The crying will not stop. Grief has me by the throat.

In the weeks that follow I go through all James's old stuff. His papers; completed and half-completed scripts; notes he has written to me. His presence is everywhere. This cruel contradiction between the physicality of his belongings makes him feel both tantalisingly close and unbearably far away. Steeping myself in his written words, I can almost hear his voice.

Some people are talking about him as if he has already died. Or they avoid mentioning him at all, as if fearing his disease might be contagious. Like some scary voodoo mask, dementia stalks them.

My doctor prescribes antidepressants and sleeping tablets. I take them for a couple of weeks but hate the way they deaden me, making me feel my pain through a dense fog. So I stop taking them, knowing I have to go through this, feel every emotion. The pain is my punishment for putting James into a care home.

There are moments when I cannot help feeling it would have been better for him – and me – if I had put him in a coffin. At least that would have had some sort of dignity about it, a proper ending. Then I am overwhelmed with guilt that the thought even enters my head.

Good friends are trying to distract me by inviting me to dinner, the cinema, the theatre. It's not working.

Colette asks me to go with her to her old friend's wedding in Vienna. I know she's wanting to pull me out of the bog of insanity. She and Brigid, Maureen, and my much loved aunt Ann, tell me over and over again, 'You must live, get your life back. You must do it for James. It's what he would have wanted.'

I don't want to accept their words. I don't want to

understand them. I'm drowning in my deep ocean of pain but they won't let me. They don't give up, despite my rejection of them.

In the past James's mantra on life, which he had said so often, had always been, Carpe Diem. But I'm not ready to hear that now.

* * *

Vienna isn't working. I watch the guests dancing to Strauss and all I want is James here dancing with me. My last visit to Vienna was on our honeymoon so it is little wonder I'm thinking of him all the time. All I can think is 'James will never visit Vienna again, the city and home of Mozart, the composer he so loved.'

I start to reach out to dementia helplines. I sound like a child sobbing down the line: 'I'm not coping ...'. I'm having trouble finding someone who understands. They're kind, but most of them are the adult children of dementia patients in their eighties. How can they possibly know how it feels to lose someone to the disease who's only fifty-eight? James and I don't have children. It's always been just him and me, and we've been everything to each other.

But they're all kind, these people manning the helplines, although they tell me not to hope for a miracle cure, and they don't profess to have any quick-fix solutions. One eighty-year-old spouse spoke to me about grief. 'It's like climbing the Eiger,' she told me. 'You just have to get through it day by day and deal with it yourself. The best cure of all is to make a new life.'

I try to find solace in nature but that's not working either. I get into the car with Mouse and drive miles out into the countryside. Mouse has a lovely time chasing rabbits while I sit on a fence and cry. I stay till the crows caw their way home and hear a curlew mournfully call as he flies overhead. I leave before my thoughts overwhelm me as I look back on my life with James. Exhausted, I return home.

It feels like there is no escape. At night I'm tormented by manic dreams. In one dream I'm queueing up with a line of lambs in an abattoir waiting to be slaughtered. As it comes to my turn I accept it, because I am one of a flock and at least we are all together. In another I'm swimming in a sea desperate to get to the shore. As I swim towards it, it appears to be further away than I expected. Exhausted I wake in a terrifying sweat.

The thought of suicide hovers over me like a black raven. I've planned how to do it. I'm saving the sleeping and antidepressant tablets the doctor so generously gave me. They're stacked in the bathroom cupboard. I plan to take them with James's favourite bottle of Montrachet wine.

In my saner moments the thought of abandoning James stops me. Who would know and care for him in the way I do? Who would visit him and bring his favourite things to eat? Who would check that he is being looked after properly?

'I'm here for the long haul James, and will accompany you as you trundle down your isolated, lonely path, on your long trek through this terrible journey called dementia. Of course I am.'

15 : Visiting Time

*She stood there in the storm, and when the wind did not blow her
way she adjusted her sails. – Elizabeth Edwards*

My first visit to see James arrives. Sara had said that I
needed to stay away for the first few weeks in order
to let him settle in, and it's been desperately hard not being
able to see him.

I enter his room and when he sees me he gives me the
broadest smile and holds out his arms for a hug. In tears, I
fall into them.

Seeing my James living in this new alien place,
surrounded by dementia patients, is heart wrenching. He is
so utterly vulnerable.

It's soon clear that dementia has claimed even more of
him. As we sit in the dining room he seems so vulnerable
among all the other residents. He can't lift a fork or a glass
to his mouth now, let alone string a sentence together. He
doesn't know who he is or even where he is.

'James, where the hell are you? What would I give to
have you back just for a day.'

I sit with him for hours looking through photographs of
his past. The ones on the walls show him filming on

location, going to award ceremonies, on holiday with me. Will they trigger some reminder in his mind of his old life and our years together?

He stares at the images for hours. Sometimes he smiles and points at a photo – filming in America and Africa; skiing in France; fly fishing on a loch; pets we have loved and lost. He laughs and says, 'Me, you, me. Love love, love, me, fuck, fuck, fuck.'

My heart breaks for what he's lost, for what we have lost and will never have again.

Going through this horrible time is hell. I drown in the sadness of it all.

I become more protective of him. Now he is my incomprehensible child. This gorgeous, once so talented man is lost to me for ever. No more long chats. No more fun, no more laughter, no more life. I have to accept that I will never be able to reach him again, nor will he ever be able to reach me.

My heart breaks with every visit. I try to be normal on the outside, but inside I continue in a crazed mess, desperately trying to fight off mini mental breakdowns. Hardest of all are his continued chats to me in a language I cannot fully understand.

Whatever he says, even if it makes no sense at all, I grasp at the words eagerly. But in the weeks that follow his language skills become even more impaired. Trying to follow the continuous chat in a language I can't understand becomes nigh on impossible.

'Just us no one in world ... us nobody nobody say well it's great ... nobody gets us ... beautiful things of that other ... things say I'm first of this both of them better than me ... me to you me would be great never told them ... shit shit ... just me you ... nobody seems me ... that's the way ... it's great on that ... believe ... it see sure ... everything out ... it's easy ... up there ... keep that it ... make sure of it ... all day all time ... all bloody everything that's good ... beautiful ... great ... love it ... I know ... love love love love.'

I try desperately to grasp the gist of it. I am certain he has an awareness that he is not where he should be, and through his fast-diminishing 'window' he is trying to say to me, 'I want you and me to get out of this fucking care home and for us to be together.' He's angry at strangers intruding on his life; only 'us' matters. And he 'loves, loves, loves me.'

Over the next days and weeks I watch James interact – or not – with the staff at the care home. He tends to view all carers of any shape or size with suspicion. As far as he is concerned they are intruding on his life, uninvited. He refuses to let them come anywhere near him and swears at them, telling them to 'bugger off'. He detests the smell of their perfume. He dislikes some more than others.

They tell me he took off his slipper and tried to hit one of them. It's like he's a child who, when mother isn't there, does all sorts of naughty things, but when I arrive all tantrums disappear. I get the smile and the gentleness and cooperation. And so far he's letting me do anything – bath him, change his soiled clothes, trim his hair, cut his nails. I find doing his personal care preserves the closeness between us, and for a second I can pretend this is all a terrible dream and I'll wake up and everything will be as it was before.

Sometimes he seems more restless than at other times. I remember the tiny 'window' of knowing, which is characteristic of Pick's Disease. At these times I think the window is a little wider than the experts predicted, and knowing how highly intelligent James is, I guess he feels more than any of us can understand.

He points at the main exit door, indicating he wants to get out of 'fucking this fuck place.' I walk him into the garden but once he's there he looks around confused as if he doesn't know why he wanted to get out in the first place.

Looking at the other care home residents, I can't help noticing how compliant many of them are compared to James.

One, a retired naval officer, stands in the large sitting room gazing through the bay windows across the car park, legs astride, feet apart, one hand on hip, the other shielding his eyes, saying endlessly: 'Bit choppy out there today eh? There's a fine swell.'

Barbara, a retired headmistress, walks her pupils, 'dolls', in a pram every morning.

George, a former dentist, tells me, 'I met your father yesterday. We had a great chat'.

Jenny tells me, 'I took my car in for a service this afternoon and I'm going to the theatre this evening.' Beautifully dressed and very articulate, it took me several visits to realise she had dementia. Many appear to be content in their twilight world, oblivious to life going on around them.

Bonnie is one of those, with this more benign form of dementia. She wanders into James's room and sits on his bed. She looks at the photographs on his wall and chats in a nonsensical way, saying, 'Yes it is. I know it. Yes it is. I know it can be.' And she smiles.

There is Tom, who is in the early stages of dementia. His wife Alice is devoted to him, constantly fussing around him and offering soothing words. She tells me, 'Despite all the changes in Tom I'm still enjoying his wit and humour before he deteriorates. It's what I love the most'.

The saddest of all is Kate, who is in her early sixties. Her husband Rod, despairingly, could not accept her late stage Alzheimer's and chose to walk away. He was unable to live with the disease that robbed him of life's memories, and their companionship and intimacy. He found it impossible to live with the helplessly vacant, repetitious conversation, violent and incontinent wife who did not recognise him any more. She was not the girl he married.

We were chatting one day and he broke down as he told

me, 'Our daily life was imploding because of the way she behaved. Her mood swings. It's a living death.' Unable to cope mentally and physically, and torn with guilt, he felt he had no choice but to walk away. I later found out he had filed for divorce.

* * *

As the months go by I find I am becoming more accepting of James being in the care home. But at the same time I am finding it more and more difficult to come to terms with the fact that his speech is now almost entirely gone.

My James, once so brilliantly articulate, is now reduced to single syllable words. I had been warned he would lose the ability to utter even a word. The thought of never hearing that beautiful voice again is a nightmare. This bloody disease is not going to spare me anything. It was out to take every last vestige of what was left of him and leave nothing in its wake. Was there no end to this sadistic bastard? There was definitely no end to my heartbreak.

More strange behaviour emerges. James has taken to wearing two ties. This is the man who always hated to wear even one, and only ever did so grudgingly for a formal event. Friends and carers laugh at his new look, especially as the ties are worn with a shirt over a white T-shirt, together with a baseball cap.

Even after so many years of living with James's

dementia, I'm no closer to understanding the strange and faulty wiring of his brain, and what is likely to happen next. As the situation worsens it's taking over my life. With absolutely no professional support – no-one at all monitoring his or my journey as they would, for instance, a cancer or Parkinson's patient – I am entirely alone. The nightmare has moved in with me permanently.

My heart breaks with every visit. In this world of dementia we continue to exist – me watching for any little sign of cognition, James showing only that tiny 'window'. But it's enough to make him aware that something bad is happening to him and that, like an animal at the slaughterhouse, he's moving inexorably towards the stun gun.

Does he have any memory left? I'm not sure. I play him all the music he loves – Mozart, Verdi, Leonard Cohen, Chris Rhea, Fleetwood Mac. Anything that might reach him and bring him closer to me. Sometimes he smiles, but is he enjoying the sounds? I sit with him for hours as he turns the pages of the picture books that I buy for him. He stares for a very long time at a picture and it is as if his scrambled brain is desperately trying to decipher who or what it is about.

One particular photograph, a Scottish landscape, becomes his obsession. Why, I'm not sure. Does it mean something to him? We've never been to Scotland together, never talked about it. But does this photo trigger some far-off memory from his childhood, long before he met me, perhaps?

I'll never know.

I bring him tasty food to eat. Slices of roast lemon chicken, his favourite fruit cake. I put seasonal flowers in his room in the hope that the bright colours and scent will trigger a memory.

I wait patiently for signs.

* * *

As time passes I feel myself thinking more and more of what this is doing to me, Nula. I am no longer the artist who was brought in to depict Early Man in Africa. As well as that I spent time in South Africa, teaching art to the children in Soweto. I also worked with Aborigines in Australia. I was an established painter and sculptor; I worked with Henry Moore. Later I became an interior designer with projects all over the world. I worked not only in Ireland, but also London, Paris, New York, Los Angeles and Chicago. Interior Magazines published my finished work and newspapers interviewed me about my various projects. One of London's top interior design companies, with a royal connection, named a wallpaper after me, 'The Nula Stripe'.

None of that counts for anything anymore. It might as well not have existed. In the space of five years I became a full-time carer. Today I am someone else, someone I never thought I would be. I am Nula, the wife of a man with dementia.

I need to visit James every day. That is now my sole occupation. It is the only way to hold on to him, to stay close to him. I am too emotionally and physically exhausted to try to restart any aspect of my old life.

My self-confidence – along with my bank balance – is being steadily eroded. The huge care home fees force me to sell my last and only home, a small cottage I was renovating in the west of Ireland. I intended doing a book on the renovation using my skills as a designer. But it's impossible to continue as the care home costs escalate, and there's not a thing I can do about it.

My friends and family have stopped asking about James. It's simply that they don't know what to do or say to me anymore. They can't hold on indefinitely, forever asking, 'How is he?'

One friend went so far as to say to me, 'I'm bloody sick of seeing you living and talking about dementia and what it's doing to you. You've got to move on and make a life for yourself.'

Although I dread the visits, I cannot stay away. He is still my darling James and the longing to see him never ceases, not even when there is no glimmer of recognition in his beautiful green eyes.

'Do you know me, James?'

No response.

But then there's a sudden smile, and it's enough to sustain me for that moment.

Invariably, after I leave him, I routinely sneak back to see if he realises I'm gone. I watch him engrossed in his photograph book, oblivious to my absence. In one way that is a small comfort; in another, it only compounds my sadness.

16 : A Friend in Need

*Friendship is born at that moment when one person
says to another, 'What! You too?' – C.S. Lewis*

In the weeks and months that follow I carry on in a
zombie state. I have no interest or desire to do anything.
I am emotionally bankrupt.

One day I come across an injured fox lying on waste
ground. It makes no attempt to run away when I approach.
It looks helpless. I get water and dog food and place it close.
It does not move. It is obvious the fox has been injured and
is in a lot of pain. It mirrors how I feel. My heart breaks at
the sight of it. I telephone the RSPA. They examine the little
fox and tell me, 'It appears to have been hit by a car and
probably has internal injuries. We'll have to put it down.' I
sobbed and sobbed. It was too much. How I wished they
could have injected me and put me out of my misery and
sent me into oblivion.

I had to get help. I was going insane.

In a chance encounter with a friend, counselling was
suggested: 'I think it might help you to talk about James, his
loss and your living and coping without him, and help you
to move on with a new life.' I nodded. I was desperate to

navigate my way out of this hell and maybe a counsellor would provide a map to find a way through. I arrived at her clinic and the first thing she did was hug me. I broke down and sobbed. I discovered she was an ex-nun and married to an ex-monk. She was full of compassion and an enormous help in getting me to accept my situation and move forward. Unfortunately, the sessions ended two months later when she left with her husband and moved to Scotland.

* * *

John arrived on the scene at precisely the right time, and from the moment I met him he became a lifeline when I was feeling myself sinking. Some people in my life did rise to the challenge brilliantly and I'm so grateful to those who tried to understand and help. Some ran for the hills, of course, and that's just the way of things. Fear of madness is even worse that fear of cancer, and dementia is one big taboo. People do tend to evaporate when they see the white chalk cross on the door.

The best sort of friend has to be the one who is experiencing the same thing in their lives, and this is how it was with John. He knew how it was, what I would be feeling – because he had felt the same. It was, good, too, to be able to accept help and give it in return, not to be feeling a drain on someone else who was helping through the goodness of their heart. John needed me; I needed him. It was symbiosis.

Out of the blue, Sara telephones me.

'I've decided to give a lunch for all the spouses and relatives. I think it would be great if you could meet each other.' She adds that she is especially thinking of me, knowing I've been hit particularly hard. 'It might be a comfort to you, Nula. You can talk about what you've been going through with others who've been through the same.'

She tells me that there's one man in particular she'd like me to meet. 'John, Bonnie's husband. Like you, he's not coping all that well.' She didn't pause for breath, as if sensing my hesitancy. 'He's got a similar background to James. He's worked in television too. I reckon you might have a lot in common.'

I think of Bonnie, the compliant, gentle patient two doors up from James. I've got to know her quite well in the time he's been in the home. As soon as she sees me in the corridor she usually walks up to me and says something like, 'I knew you would come.' I say, 'Hello Bonnie,' giving her a gentle hug. She gives a shudder and smiles, lifting her arms up to cover her chest as she giggles nervously.

She often wanders in and sits on James's bed just listening to our chatter and smiling. She looks at the pictures on the wall and smiles, saying 'Is nice, nice '. She helps herself to his chocolates on the top of his chest of drawers. She takes a handful and eats them casually in front of him.

Sometimes I take her and James to the coffee shop and get her a cup of hot chocolate, her favourite. She is always cold, and gives a shiver to show me she is, so I'll know to wrap a pashmina around her.

She has a strange and ethereal beauty and loves to dance to the music played by the entertainer who comes in to play the piano in the residents' lounge. She moves to the ABBA, Frank Sinatra and Vera Lynn songs, waving her arms, oblivious to all around her.

When I turn on the CD player in her room and she sings along to one of her old favourites, it brings tears to my eyes:

'I'll be seeing you

In all the old familiar places

That this heart of mine embraces

All the way ...'

We have similar colouring, she and I, and new staff often ask, 'Are you and Bonnie related?'

It's strange that in all these months I've never bumped into her husband.

Almost all the guests at the lunch Sara has invited me to are the adult children of elderly parents with dementia. This means that they and I do not have much in common. Losing one's parents is an accepted part of life, but losing one's spouse is not.

As soon as I'm introduced to John it is different. And as he describes his own feelings of loss and heartbreak it is as if a light has been switched on in my soul; when he reaches out to me there is an instant recognition and connection.

It was as if he was desperate to tell me his story and share his sad experience.

'I've got to know James very well while visiting Bonnie. She likes to wander in and out of his room and look at the photographs on his wall. Bonnie was diagnosed three years ago. She was the love of my life. It's been hell going through it and heart wrenching to see her here in this alien place. We had made so many plans before dementia claimed her. To see her going further and further away from me just rips me apart. The heartbreak is beyond words. No one prepared me for the pain of losing her to dementia. It's been my worst nightmare.'

He talked on, as if he needed to share it with someone going through the same pain. 'We first met over thirty years ago. I guess we were lucky to have had twenty-five wonderful years together.'

In between courses, our conversation was interrupted by the other guests sitting around the table relaying their stories about losing their spouses and parents. It was as if we were all released from an emotional prison, and desperate to tell our story, and the talking and the sharing was a necessary route and a huge help in liberating us. Whilst I could feel their pain and sympathise with them, none of their stories touched me in the way John's did. His heartbreak mirrored my experience exactly and described the same feeling of loss I felt. There was an instant recognition and an instant connection. It was as if he had reached out to me. I could not explain it logically. All I knew was, I had to respond and find out more.

I was taken aback by the similarities in our situations. His was identical to mine. His wife was a few years older than James, in her late sixties. But the comfort was that he had described the same feelings of despair and loss of hope that I felt. It was a huge connection, and an enormous consolation to know that there was someone who was not only in the same situation as me and going through what I was going through, but feeling exactly as I was. He, like me, was younger, and he described having to deal with the dreaded dementia and trying to live with it and through it, in exactly the way I was.

Suddenly, I wasn't the only spouse travelling down this lonely, desolate and isolated path of living and dealing with dementia.

An avalanche of questions poured out of me: How are you coping? Do you have any support? How have you accepted the finality of the diagnosis? Do you have any miracle cure for getting through the pain of it? How are you filling the void of her absence?

I have a million 'hows'.

It is very unusual for me to reach out to a complete stranger, but heartbreak is infecting every part of my life in the cruellest way: I am not coping and I don't care who knows it.

Had he been a woman I would have wanted the same. The desperation to share is all that matters, to know that there's someone out there who is going through the same as me.

* * *

Spring has arrived and I visit James, feeling acutely his lack of awareness or joy in the changing of the season, the budding plants and the birdsong. Each day on my arrival, I search for him in a maze of corridors, which he walks endlessly as though trying to find a way out. Then I see his tall frame. No outstretched arms any more, although he smiles and chatters in his 'non-sense' way. I hug him.

If the sun is shining I lead him into the garden linking his arm. I point out the flowering trees and plants; pick a flower and hold it under his nose to smell the scent. No interest at all.

For me, though, Spring comes as a relief: it brings with it a little hope and a calmer, more accepting state of mind.

* * *

Dear Nula,

It was good to meet you and talk last week at the lunch. I was struck – as you had been – by how similar our experiences are. So often, as I think I said when we chatted, people come up to me and say they understand what I'm going through, because their mother or father, grandmother or grandfather – always someone in their 80s or even 90s – has or had dementia. I want to scream at them No! You don't understand, this is my life partner, the person I had intended entering old age with, spending the rest of my life with, and hopefully dying with. Yet, little by little, all those hopes are being stripped away.

I understand totally what you say about no longer being able to share. You go out to dinner, you travel, but there is no James. Bonnie and I travelled to central Europe countless times to research books I was writing. We stayed in wonderful spa hotels, went to the opera, laughed together, shared it all. Now this is all gone.

I have tried, like you, doing it alone. Twice in the last year I have gone to Germany and done the things we loved, but this time alone. I must admit to an extent I relished the freedom. I could move at my own pace. I did not have to keep repeating what I said. But a couple of nights on my own, no one to talk to, nothing to share, was enough. I realised I am not very good at being alone – the legacy, I suppose, of more than 20 years when every experience, every thought, was shared with the woman who was the love of my life. I find myself using the past tense, because although that woman is still here living with me, the woman I knew has gone. I sense it is the same with James.

Meeting you at the lunch was a wonderful window, and

writing this email and just knowing you understand is a help. I would very much like to meet outside the care home, and talk things over more, if you would like to. It might be better to make it after the summer. I am hoping to spend most of the summer at our house in France. I will have to sell it. It's too heartbreaking to keep it now without Bonnie.

Sorry for the long email, but when you meet a kindred spirit the words kind of pour out. Again, I suspect that's something you understand.

Look forward to hearing from you, and with warmest wishes.

John.

Hello Nula,

I hope you don't mind me being in touch again.

I nipped over to Florida for a few days to see my son … When I got back I went to see Bon. When she saw me she beamed a smile and said she hadn't seen me for such a long time. But there was no recognition in her eyes. I decided to ask gently, 'Come on, make me happy, tell me my name.' 'I know who you are, don't be silly.' 'Of course you do, that's great … come on, tell me my name.' 'I'll tell you if you tell me yours,' she said. I had only been away 5 days.

It was heartbreaking there was no reaction. She looked at me and smiled again, got up and walked away from me down the corridor. I broke down and left in tears.

That evening I had to get on a stage in front of 1200

people at a black tie awards dinner for the pharmaceutical industry. I hadn't expected three massive photos of Bonnie and me projected on the wall behind – our wedding day, us at a television event and another at a concert. (I had been warned but forgot.) I walked onto the stage, saw the photos, tried to speak and couldn't. Ever seen a man choke in front of a roomful of people? I managed to pull myself together. Afterwards I died the death of a thousand hugs from more glamorous women than I have seen in a single place in my life. So I suppose it's not all bad.

France in two weeks. It really is living from one day to the next, isn't it?

There now haven't I rabbitted on. But as I've said before, there is nothing quite like talking to someone who is living through this as well. But you still don't need a mini-book like this to drop into your inbox and busy life.

John

Dear John,

Back in London. Visiting James today was so depressing. Conversation with him went something like this ... every day but shit of them ... nothing shit ... up and up ... me up ... beautiful thing ... one two fords ... first one say a connection ... know as you well ... is great ... is great on that, so beautiful ... never told them ... just me you ... nobody seems me ... that's the way ... it's great on that ... believe ... it see ... everything out, it's easy, make sure of it

... all day all that time ... all bloody everything, that's good ... out of it ... beautiful ... great ... love it ... I know ... it's great on that, me told sure of it – and on and on.

His desperation to make himself understood is heartbreaking ...

The last weeks have been hectic. I have moved into a very small apartment. We had so much stuff, I just packed it all away into storage and will sort it out when my life is more settled.

Nula

Dear Nula,

I was so pleased to get your e mail last weekend. It's been a difficult week with emotional decisions. I'm off to France crack of dawn tomorrow.

A happier thought. Are you free at all from late September? If so, would you let me buy you lunch or dinner to thank you for listening to all this stuff? It would be lovely to say a proper hello away from the care home. I somehow doubt we would be stuck for conversation ...

Dear John,

I spend August bank holiday with friends in Wiltshire. They put on an opera every year, in the grounds of their beautiful garden in aid of a local charity. Although it was welcome distraction from dementia and care homes, I was saddened that not one person mentions James.

Colette takes him out for the afternoon while I am away. She has not seen him for several weeks and is shocked to see how much dementia has taken away. She laughs when she sees him dressed in his baseball cap, two ties and a cashmere scarf on a warm summer's day. She asks him, 'What's my name, James?' But he just laughs at her and says, 'I know you ... of course I know course.' During their lunch he keeps taking out his wallet and producing his television ID cards, laying them out in a row to show her who he was. As she chats to him, Colette asks, 'Where's Nula?' He just laughs.

I am in tears when she tells me. He hasn't said my name in a long time but he still does say 'loves loves loves' when he sees me.

It doesn't get any easier does it?

It will be good to meet. The 29th suits.

Nula

Dear Nula,

Well I had my 48-hour break, flew to London to present a concert, and what a guilty pleasure it was! Moving at my own speed through the airport, just being able to concentrate on what I was doing, was a form of bliss.

On day one while I was away, phoning the care home to see how she was, Dawn the carer said they had watched my concert on television. She asked Bon, 'Do you know who that is?' Bon answered, 'I think he's famous but I don't know his name.' …

I'm really glad we've got an evening fixed. Shall we say 7:00?

Dear Nula,

… At a charity function the other day a colleague told me a friend of hers had said grief ambushes you. Isn't that perfect? Just when you least expect it, you get ambushed. It's the little things that do it – the empty chair, the single eggcup at breakfast, her favourite coat in the cupboard.

Really looking forward to meeting you for dinner, chose your favourite restaurant!

Right, I'm off to find the corkscrew.

John

17 : Tentative Steps

In the midst of winter, I found at last there was, within myself, an invincible summer. – Albert Camus

Our dinner turns out to be awkward and our conversation turns into a bit of a tennis match. John says 'I don't want you to think I'm looking for another relationship. I'm not. I've had the best and it could never be repeated. I'm now perfectly content to be alone.' And he goes on to say, as if I haven't heard him the first time: 'What I had could never be repeated. It was beyond perfect.'

Isn't this a meeting to share the journey? Why is he laying down ground rules?

I find myself pulling back, uncomfortable. What does he think I'm looking for?

My serve. The tennis match resumes in an atmosphere of discomfort. 'I'm not looking for a relationship either. I've had the most amazing life with James and I know it can never be repeated. There will never be another James. He was unique.'

Then I talk and talk about James – how wonderful, bright and creative he was. Then stressing my point: 'He's irreplaceable.'

I say to John that all I want is to share with someone who's in the same situation as me, nothing more, and that had he been a woman I would have done exactly the same, and met her for the same reasons.

He looks at me, surprised. 'Would you really?'

'Yes, yes I would.'

He'd not expected that.

It surprises me when John takes out his diary at the end of the evening and says, casually, 'Shall we do this again?'

We agree to meet in a few weeks.

The next day he texts me. 'Carpe diem, and let's take one friggin' day at a time.'

It is as if James is talking to me. It's exactly the language he would have used.

* * *

In Florida I meet the estate agents and our Florida house is on the market. I hated having to sell this piece of paradise, but with James in care and not working full time, it's not feasible for me to hold on to it any longer. And coming here alone, with the many memories it evokes of good times gone, only adds to the sadness. The deed is done, and part of me feels heartbroken all over again.

I walk through our beautiful home across the pale ivory limestone floor, seeing my watercolours of shells and boats on the walls amidst the shelves and shelves of books. It feels strange not to have James here.

We used to come every winter to escape the madness of Christmas and the January cold. We'd swim and cycle or walk along the beach collecting shells which now lie on the lanai deck outside. We'd sprawl on the bleached linen sofas losing ourselves in American novels or catching up on films we'd missed, whilst outside in the searing heat the fish jumped in the creek.

Losing the house; losing you, losing the life we had. It feels like heartbreak upon heartbreak.

I stay on for several weeks and enjoy the warm sunshine. I doubt I will ever return once the sale has gone through. But it's good too, being here.

One afternoon I'm out cycling, and a nice old gentleman walking along the path sees me and calls out, 'Oh my, you do make a bike look good!'

It brings the biggest smile to my face.

Dear Nula,
You seem to have a sixth sense about when to text. In tube on way out to Sundial, depressed, mobile beeped, and I thought wouldn't that be nice if it was Nula, thought it won't be, n guess what! Instant smile. J

John keeps in touch with emails. It was good to have someone who cared and understood and I enjoyed having a friendship again.

The searing isolation of my life without James compelled me to see John. We continued to meet every four weeks or so. We attended operas, concerts, music recitals, theatres and the cinema. We treasured those times and relished the sharing, even more so because of what we had lost. In between, we visited James and Bonnie. Early in our friendship neither of us questioned or analysed our situation. We had not thought beyond meeting as two people going through the same loss and sharing the journey. We just accepted the need to meet and appreciate the companionship and comfort it brought us.

We didn't expect or ask anything from each other. It was as if something within us knew that this was the only way – the only route to getting through the horrendous loss of James and Bonnie. We enjoyed and made the most of what we had found, in each other.

Travelling to see James my heart would be full of foreboding. The contradiction of desperately wanting to see him, to be near him yet dreading it at the same time, always hit me. As soon as I entered his room, the sight of him overwhelmed me with sadness. He was there physically, but was long gone mentally. I would sit with him for hours but could tell him nothing of where I had been or what I had done. My life was just me now, no more sharing. Nor was I able to ask him how he was, or what he was thinking behind that blank stare as he looked out beyond me into the distance. A wall of silence called Dementia was now erected

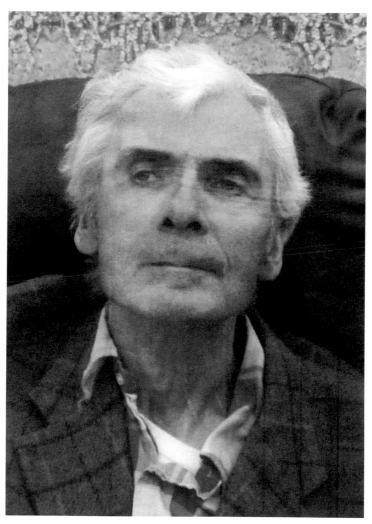

James in 2013, eight years into dementia

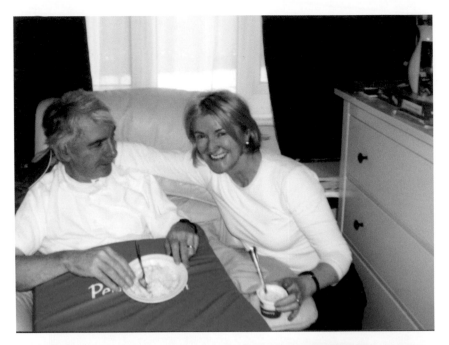

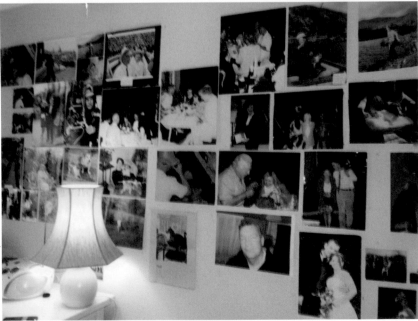

Top. Visiting James at the care home, 2012
Bottom: Photographs hoping to keep the memories alive on the wall of James's room

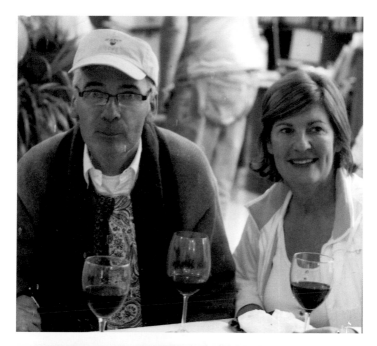

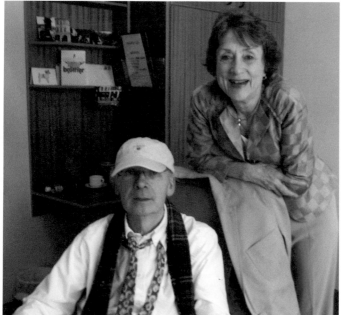

Top. Dressed in two ties and baseball cap for a lunch date with Colette
Bottom: James with his former wife, Dame Carol Black

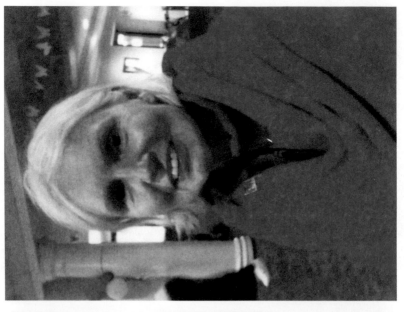

James in his final months at the care home, 2014

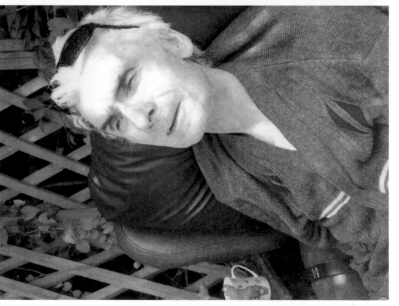

Bonnie soon after going into care, 2010

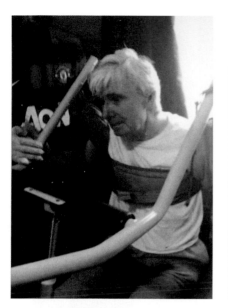
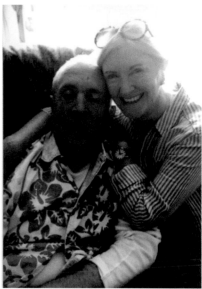
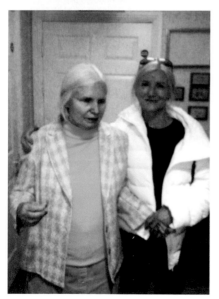
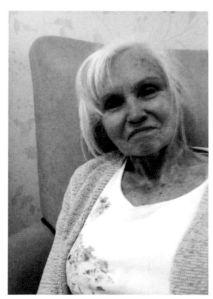

From top left: James struggling with the hoist in the care home, 2012; my friend Mona's darling husband Phil Fisher, together with James and Bonnie The Trinity, 2012; Taking Bonnie into the garden, 2013; Bonnie before her fall, 2014

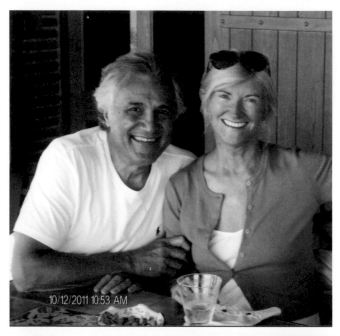

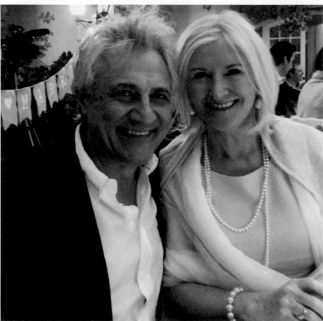

Top. First holiday with John in Greece - not a total success
Bottom. In France, 2014, attending my niece Nia's wedding
to Arthur

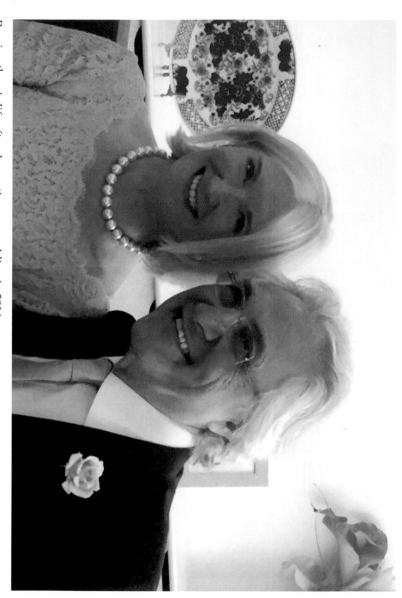

Proving there's life after dementia, our wedding in 2016

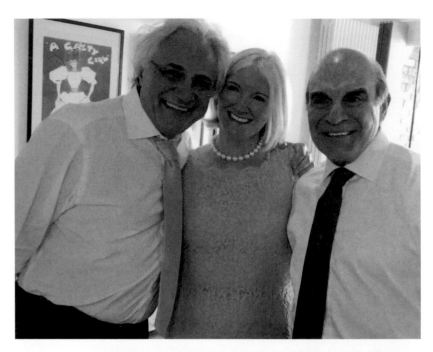

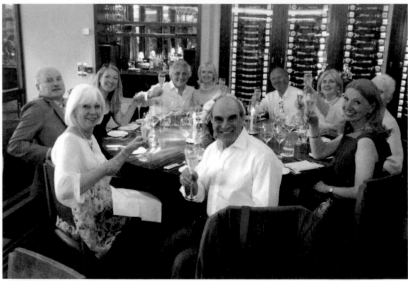

Top. John and Nula, with John's brother David
Bottom. A small intimate wedding dinner

so high between us that neither of us would never ever be able to reach the other again.

But even though I dreaded the visits, I continued. I could not stay away. The longing to see him and be near him never went away.

18 : Uncertain Times

Guilt is a rope that wears thin – Ayn Rand

John and I meet in the coming months, we share, talk endlessly about James and Bonnie and the care home staff and life going on around us. We are in a bizarre situation – how are we to deal with the fact that we are both still married to two people, now far beyond our reach, living in a care home?

When I'm with James I long to ask him, 'What should I do? My life without you is a mess. I'm not sure who or what I am, or where I'm going.'

In the past he would have advised or helped me when my life veered off course. Now I feel rudderless.

I remind myself that he always told me, 'If anything happens to either one of us the other must go out and find a new life.'

But it doesn't change the fact that I'm not sure I even want to.

Hell – we make it through to Christmas!

It is such a help having John. We meet up at the care home on Boxing Day and join in the jolly singalong. Then again on New Year's Eve, when we raise our glasses and drink to James and Bonnie. When Big Ben chimes midnight we hug each other and agree it's the best New Year either of us has had in seven years.

* * *

Then Vienna again, and it's no better. This time John invites me to join him for a weekend to hear Wagner's The Flying Dutchman. I am suffused with past memories of the freezing cold December of my and James's honeymoon – so cold that when we returned to our hotel James lovingly ran a bath for me, putting in the scented oils and swirling the oily water, and as I slipped into it he massaged my whole body to warm me. It was such an intimate time.

Now I'm here with a man I hardly know. Pangs of guilt climb onto my shoulder and sit there for the whole weekend.

* * *

Life continues in a frenzy of uncertainty. I have no permanent home to call my own, having sold ours, and have no power of attorney in place because by the time we discovered James had dementia he was deemed to be too mentally unsound to transfer any legal power to me. Our joint finances have to stay on hold until after his death, so now my money worries are mounting.

Uncertain times.

It doesn't help that I'm leading a double life: one, visiting a husband I adore but who is unable to connect with me on any level for years – who doesn't recognise or acknowledge me in any way; the other, trying to make a new life of sorts with John, who is doing his best to help me get through it (as I hope I am for him).

I long for my old secure life.

Out of the blue, my mobile rang and a voice at the other end asked,' Are you available to do some design work?" Disinterested, I let the voice continue, "It's a lovely project on an old country estate, a farmhouse and three cottages in need of complete renovation in a beautiful part of Sussex."

I decided to find out more and hearing the detail, a meeting was arranged to visit the site. The location, house and cottages, were stunning and the owners charming. Both in their mid-eighties. The estate had become too difficult for them to manage. They needed to renovate the house and the cottages to maximise their selling potential in order to realise as much capital as possible. This would give them enough money to downsize and move into more manageable sheltered accommodation. It would allow them to live their remaining years in financial security and comfort.

I decided there and then to do it. My life would have a purpose, albeit a small one. Could this give a kick start and a new direction to my life? It certainly was a distraction from dementia. In the coming weeks I worked alongside the architect and the builders. I loved every minute. The old adrenalin kicked in and I was in creative heaven.

Alone in the evenings I found myself in country bliss, surrounded by acres of green fields, woods, wild animals. I had plenty of time to think back on the last nine years, how dementia had not only stolen my James but had stolen my life as well.

Yet I marvelled at how fate had found a way to get me through. Yes, I was living a new life, and it helped hugely to have John as a friend to share the journey.

Here in the little cottage they had installed me in I started to feel a new 'me' emerging. I felt renewed and was becoming a more contented self.

I returned to London at the weekend to see John, but it interrupted my recovery. We attended a smart lunch party, hosted by a work colleague of his I had only met once. The temperature on the riverside terrace was searingly hot. I tried to show interest in an ageing actress's past life as she chatted on. She didn't have an ounce of interest in mine. The heat and the vacuous conversation around the lunch table, with a banker and other corporate guests, got to me. I noticed John's eyes following a pretty girl. It irked me. The recovery, this new life, was going to be more difficult than I imagined.

A few weeks later we went to Edinburgh to attend a

two-man play; Steven Berkoff, an actor/playwright, friend and neighbour of John's, was putting it on for the festival. During the visit, we met and had dinner with James's sister Maureen who lived there. I wanted her to meet John, who was becoming the new man in my life.

Meeting Maureen was emotional. She reminded me of James. She has his good looks and brilliant mind. I love her like a real sister. She had been an enormous support to me when James was first diagnosed with dementia. She had listened to my sobs on the telephone and carried me through in the early days. She was one of those who encouraged me to put James into professional care when dementia took over more of him. And she stood by me in the years that followed.

At the end of the evening she applauded my new life, hugged me and whispered, 'James would be so glad to see you happy. He'd want you to live and I know he'd be cheering you on.' She smiled, 'I like John, he's good for you. You're good for each other. I'm so happy you both found a way through all the pain. I know James would have liked him.'

Returning to London John said, 'I enjoyed meeting Maureen, I want to know more about your life. I want to meet your family.' Yes, I thought, that's difficult. My parents are long dead. My family are scattered through Ireland, America and Australia.

James was my life. We just had each other. We led a

nomadic lifestyle and travelled extensively. He was my present, my past and my future.

I returned to Sussex and finished the project.

* * *

James is getting increasingly difficult for the carers to handle. His general health is deteriorating dramatically, which is having a catastrophic effect on his moods. The dementia is encroaching more into the frontal lobes of his brain. That is the medical description. Put simply, he is becoming a non-person.

Not wanting to stress him further when he's abusive and difficult and refusing to be touched, the carers often leave him unshaven, without a shower, and unkempt.

I am offered an even bigger interior design project in New York, but it may as well be on the moon. I can't leave James. I need to be near enough to his care home to be able to get there by train in a few hours. The fact that he will often only allow me to bath and shave him or cut his fingernails and trim his hair prevents even the thought of going to New York.

We are having lunch in the dining room when something happens that shocks me. James leans across to another resident's plate and takes his meat with his bare hand and eats it. Oh my James, to see you reduced to this!

Bonnie too is deteriorating. She has stopped feeding

herself. Often I lean across and feed her when the carers are too busy. My regular visits have built up a sort of bond between us and she feels secure in my company. She sits in James's room when I'm visiting and remains as if she's part of our time together. She often refuses to let the carers bath her or wash her hair, but as soon as I appear and suggest: 'Bonnie, let's have a nice bath,' she repeats the same words, looking into the distance, saying, 'And so it is, yes it is,' and follows me, looking ahead and smiling.

It's a strange feeling that I am a comfort to Bonnie while I am becoming close to her husband.

Dementia is doing weird things to all of us.

19 : Like a Mistress, while a Wife

Never love unless you can
Bear with all the faults of man
— Thomas Campion

John asks me to go on holiday with him to Greece. I have never been, but encouraged by friends and family I accept with some trepidation. As soon as we arrive on the island of Samos and settle into the villa, I become even more apprehensive. How am I going to manage living in this small space with someone I've only known for a short while?

I have ample time to think on this island. Being female, my fears continue to wash in and out of my head. I knew I was going deeper and deeper into this relationship. The journey has taken me way beyond what I had expected. Would I get hurt?

He was male with male attitudes; I was female, with female neediness and emotional baggage.

Added to this, I have brought a huge suitcase full of clothes, half of which I will never wear, and for which there is nowhere near enough room in the tiny cupboard. John, predictably, has brought exactly the right amount of clothes.

There are mirrors everywhere here – a designer's trick to
make a space seem larger – and it only heightens my
insecurity. After a certain age it's better not to have mirrors
in a bedroom and when I catch sight of myself I recoil in
horror. The person who looks back at me has the face and
body of an emaciated prisoner. After seven years of caring
for James I have lost a drastic amount of weight, and in the
bright Greek sunlight I look so much older. I feel the girl
inside me vanish forever. I'm no longer twenty or forty, but
in my late fifties.

Stop, stop it! I have to stop tearing myself apart.

* * *

Living together twenty-four hours a day in a villa, I begin
to realise how much inner confidence and self-sufficiency
John has, something that only serves to heighten my own
lack of those attributes. He had a secure, happy and
comfortable childhood; mine was unsettled and
unpredictable, with a mother who managed to knock every
one of her children's self-esteem, not to mention that of my
quiet and long-suffering father.

I recall my honeymoon with James. As we left Vienna,
we got a telephone call to say my mother had collapsed at
her home in Dublin and had been rushed to hospital. It was
thought she had suffered a stroke. We drove back as quickly
as possible and arrived in Dublin to the news that it wasn't

a stroke, but an inoperable brain tumour. She was given approximately three months to live. I was shocked. This was someone who had never been ill in all the time I'd known her. Worse still, I had never been close to her.

My mother was physically a very beautiful woman, with flawless creamy skin and streaky ash blond hair. When she went to Mass on Sundays, her only social outing in this small country town community, the local men would wait outside the church just to get a glimpse of her.

I was the eldest of nine children. My mother was pregnant again a month after my birth and my younger sister was born eleven months after me. Perhaps that is why we never formed a close mother-daughter bond. I was sent to boarding school at the age of twelve. This left me with not just a huge insecurity, but a fear of abandonment too.

Confronted now by my mother's terminal illness, all my old insecurities came to the fore. Now that I had found happiness with James, there was so much I wanted to share with her.

When I arrived at the hospital, I was shocked to find an entirely new person. This was not the mother I had grown up with. It was as if the tumour had released something in her brain that had previously caused her to be unhappy, even at times unkind. But now, even terminally ill and aged seventy, here was a woman I hardly recognised, who was warm and interested in what and where I had been.

That is not to say she was incapable of acts of kindness

in years gone by. I remember once, when as children we were on a seaside holiday in the west of Ireland, she noticed a group of girls from the local orphanage being led by a nun. Without hesitation she ran across the street to the sweet shop and bought bars of chocolate for each and every one of them. We children were shocked! We had not often seen that side of her.

Now, sitting in a chair in her hospital room, she smiled and greeted me with arms outstretched, and asked, 'How was your trip, I want to hear all about it'. I hugged her and told her all about Vienna. She listened and listened. I could not believe the change in her.

A month later she died. I was pleased to have seen a very different woman at the end to the one I had known as a child, and it brought me much comfort.

James had always given me the confidence I lacked. He was reassuring, forever telling me I was talented, that nothing was too difficult for me, that I only had to try my hand at something to make a success of it.

But now I have fallen back into my old insecure self, my self-esteem is fragile, and James – my rock – is unable to put things right.

My head is bursting with questions. There is a new man in my life.

Am I being disloyal? Going out in public, with James and Bonnie in care, was still difficult for me emotionally. It was impossible for me not to think about them and where they were. I feel an awkwardness about our situation and remain unsure about how to play this new role.

John feels a little anxious too, but for different reasons. His book, My Bonnie, which he wrote before he met me, had been published. It described the heartbreak he suffered when he lost Bonnie to dementia. He was getting countrywide response to it from people with relatives suffering from dementia. They found it hugely comforting to read about his experiences, and wrote to tell him.

Despite the fact we had lived and cared for our spouses for several years, dementia had put us in an awful place. Yet we both knew we had to make a new life, it was our only way to get through the pain, sadness and the void left after losing them. No matter, it still did not assuage the guilt in either of us.

But I'm analysing too much, I have to stop. I am full of introspection – Irish introspection – the worst! Sitting out on this Greek terrace with John absorbed in his music and his book, I continued to dig into my past.

In the middle of the holiday I get a call from the care home. 'I'm afraid James had a bad fall early this morning. We're not sure how it happened but we think he stumbled getting out of bed. We took him to Watford General Hospital and he needed stitches for a nasty gash on his forehead. The casualty doctor checked him carefully and he's okay now. We'll keep a close eye on him so don't worry.'

Even my daily calls to the care home matron, who always reassures me that James is doing well and walking around in great form, don't manage to remove the 'big G' that triumphantly sits on my shoulder and refuses to leave.

The reality is that there are four of us in this relationship, and not for one moment are we allowed to forget or lose sight of that.

Sitting on the terrace on this idyllic Greek island, I am drowning in self-doubt. My past follows me. I cannot flick it away. I look back into my childhood, and replay the memories, my parents crumbling marriage, my mother's disinterest in me and my siblings; going away to boarding school; and the loneliness and isolation I felt. I detested the strict the oppressive convent rules.

I had a free spirit. That was soon knocked out of me by the nuns. The first thing the new girls in my class were asked to do was to show any talent we might have. My talent was for dancing and playing the piano. I did both, and uninhibited was pleased to be able to show what I could do.

The next day, one of the nuns, an appalling woman by the name of Mother Mercedes, met me in the corridor and said: 'What a spectacle you made of yourself. I never want to see that again. Your brains are in your feet.'

The same nun humiliated and upset me even further. In a lesson she asked me to stand up and recite a G.K. Chesterton poem, 'When Fishes Flew'. I knew it off by heart.

I loved this poem, which describes the humble donkey, looked down upon by all, which gets his moment when he is chosen to carry Jesus through Jerusalem.

I stood up to recite it. I managed the first verse, but then my stammer got the better of me. The word 'Monstrous' came out as 'M-m-m-m...'

Mother Mercedes shouted, 'Sit down you stupid girl!'

I was hurt to the core. I was thirteen years of age. In fact during the rest of the lesson I actually wrote out the poem in full from memory and put it on her desk at the end of the lesson. She ignored me and my impudence and never made another mention of it.

To this day, more than half a century later, I still wince at the memory of how that woman humiliated me. The scars have never fully healed.

Then, out of the blue two English nuns with smiling faces, visited the school with the intention of recruiting girls as novices to enter their order and work overseas as missionaries. They described the wonderful colours of Africa and India, the wonderful people and exotic animals. I volunteered immediately. It had to be more exciting and freeing than the narrow minded, restrictive life of an Irish convent boarding school. The thought of travelling to foreign parts appealed to my curious and adventurous side.

Four months later I was on a boat to England with a pot of homemade jam and a five pound note.

* * *

I loved my two years living in a convent outside Oxford. But it was not long before the doubts began and I came to the conclusion that the life of a nun was not for me. It was a blind ambition. I thought their rules of silence and fasting were unnatural and bore no relevance to God. An old Benedictine priest, who lectured us on Theology and Philosophy, and had come to know me, said, 'There's a bigger, more fun world out there for you to explore. I think it would suit you better. I don't think you're cut out to be a nun.'

I knew he was right. As I left the convent, an elderly nun hugged me and reminded me, 'Although you have left your plough in the middle of the field – our door will always be open to you.'

* * *

My connection with John is marred by the knowledge of his gloriously perfect past life with his adored Bonnie who was a much-loved only daughter. How could I ever live up to his perfect goddess? I guess I'm wanting emotional reassurance, but it's way too early for that.

Next evening at dinner, over a glass of wine, I ask him a typical, silly, girly question – and as soon as it is out of my mouth I know I shouldn't have done so.

'How do you feel about 'us'?'

My mind and my feelings are all over the place. I don't know where this relationship is going or even if I want it to go anywhere. But I'm not comfortable with it being just a casual fling and I am looking for some kind of reassurance.

Being female means I am instantly in an emotional quicksand; and being a man, he responds in an honest, male way: 'Let's take this slowly. I don't want to be hurt again. Losing Bonnie has devastated me. I never want to go through that pain again. Not letting myself fall in love too quickly is the best way to protect myself.'

I am not expecting this response. I have been naïve to assume that we have much more than this.

Outside the restaurant he puts his arm around me and whispers, 'Let's just live in the now and take one day at a time.'

I am silent. I want to cry but I can't.

* * *

Our relationship is under strain. We decide to leave the island. The basic facilities were crude, the lack of storage and smallness of the villa were oppressive in the August heat. John suggests a week in a luxury hotel in Athens.

We board a ferry a few days later in the early morning. Sitting up on deck, the cool sea air is a welcome relief from the oppressive heat of the island. We sail past the small islands with their whitewashed houses and terracotta tiled roofs, fishing boats moored in the harbours. I am struck by the beauty of Greece. Time appears to have stood still here. I envy the inhabitants and their seemingly contented lives.

We arrive in Athens and enter the modern hotel with all the comforts of air conditioning, a large bedroom and proper bathroom.

Our relationship has become decidedly chilly. Sitting by the pool John suggests lunch. Waiting for our meal to arrive an elderly Greek man walks past our table and stops. He reaches out and gently pats my head saying, 'What a lovely couple you make.' Little does he know how fragile we are. But we cannot help looking at each other and smiling at the irony of what he has said.

I suggest we get out and see Athens and its surroundings. Two days later we take a taxi to Delphi. In the shadow of Mount Parnassus lies the site of the ancient Oracle. We climb the steep hillside to Apollo's temple. On the way up John feels faint and has to sit down to get his breath. I joke that I might have to trade him in for a younger man. We both laugh and I am relieved the ease seems to have returned to our relationship.

I make a wish when we get there, as is the custom: 'I hope my friendship with John will continue.'

It isn't until a year later that I discover what John wished:

'Je veux vivre avec ma chère Nuli jusqu'à la fin de ma vie.'

* * *

When we return from Greece, my absence has made me want to see James all the more. It is as if, by some miracle, the old James, as I knew him, will greet me.

I find him in the dining room, alone, looking into space, holding a spoon, with his breakfast cereal spilt all down the front of his jumper and onto his trousers. I see the black scar on his forehead from his fall. My heart breaks at the sight of him.

I kneel on the floor in front of his chair and take his hands in mine, looking straight into his eyes, searching. 'Jamesie, it's me, your Nuli.' He smiles and mumbles some incoherent words. I repeat it over and over again: 'Jamesie, it's your Nuli, love, love, love you.' He smiles. I wrap my arms around him and his body is unresponsive.

When the carers help me to lift James out of his chair I notice immediately that his ability to walk has worsened. His feet can't work out what to do, how to put one in front of the other. Once back in his room he collapses into his chair. The short walk has exhausted him.

I put on *La Traviata*, a much loved favourite, Sutherland and Pavarotti singing Un di Felice, and the aria fills the room. In the past it would have brought James to tears. Now either he can't hear it or it means nothing to him.

* * *

Meanwhile I have a feeling that somehow I am intruding on Bonnie's life.

John has moved into a new flat. Understandably he has filled it with items they both knew – her Portmeirion china, her lamps, her vases, her wooden plaque with 'Bonnie's Kitchen' above the door. There are photographs of her in her youth, including a portrait taken in an American photographic studio when she graduated from Cornell University aged twenty-one.

Having played such a large part in his life it was inevitable that John would fill his flat with reminders of their years together. But I still feel that her ghost is following me everywhere.

At first I'm silent about my discomfort. I try to ignore the shrine to his wife's memory. I understand more than anyone his need to hold onto the past. It is all he has left of her, and his wanting to keep the memories of her alive is his only comfort.

I want to run away. I probably should. But the awful fear of facing dementia alone compels me to stay.

The strange thing is that I feel like a mistress. I am having a relationship with someone who, whilst not living with his wife, still sees her as very much a part of his life. And I feel I cannot compete with her or come anywhere close to her perfection.

With my emotions in turmoil I tell John that I've made up my mind that we should stop seeing each other. I admit to feeling it difficult with Bonnie's life all around me. 'I feel I'm treading on her past.'

He is shocked, stunned. After a few moments he says that he had no idea it was affecting me so much and he realises that he has been insensitive. Suddenly he shouts, 'You're right! I just didn't think.' Then the words tumble from him in a torrent:

'What does it matter? You saved me, we've saved each other. I want you in my life every second, every minute – no matter what. You're worth everything to me. I can't be without you. We are more than friends. We are a couple, and – more importantly – I didn't dare tell you this, but I realised very early in our friendship that you meant much more to me than I was willing to admit. I love you very much and want you in my life forever.'

We cry and hug.

Days later, he dismantles the shrine and gives most of Bonnie's possessions and her large portrait photographs to her sons. Now, on his side table is a framed photo of him and Bonnie at an awards ceremony. Next to it is a photo of James and myself attending a similar function.

* * *

Sometimes the sadness after a visit to James's home lingers for days. Our past is packed away in boxes and is in storage. I look at what's left, the photographs on his wall, and the memories come flooding in. When they do, an arrow of pain can pierce me, quite suddenly, and the bruise stays with me for a while.

One picture in particular does this to me, and yet I cannot remove it from the wall – nor do I want to. It was taken one Christmas when we were driving through France. James suddenly pulled over to the side of the country road, got out of the car and climbed over a ditch. He returned with a huge bunch of mistletoe, held it over my head and kissed me. It was so James. The photograph is of him holding the mistletoe.

The image stays with me all the way home and the sadness moves in with me and stays for days.

20 : Sentenced to a Non-Life

Love bade me welcome, yet my soul drew back – George Herbert

By the end of 2013 our relationship has moved into a better and more secure place. We have met each of our families, siblings, grandchildren. Old friends have 'celebrated our luck' at meeting each other. My friend Colette is especially thrilled that I've found a new life after James. She had watched me as I cared for James over many years, when she'd pick me up from his care home to drive me back to London, and seen me sob all the way.

Yet dementia remains with me. No matter what life I try to lead or how much I 'get on' with living, I still feel a constant, helpless frustration at not being able to relieve James from his relentless deterioration. Often I wish I could put him out of his miserable existence. Am I some cruel, heartless, sadistic bitch? No, it is so heart wrenching to watch James and Bonnie lose all semblance of basic human dignity, and beyond heartbreaking to watch them struggle to hang on to their miserable and pointless lives. They had no enjoyment in anything anymore. Their lives now were staring out into an abyss of no life.

Out of the blue an old friend calls me to tell me her Cairn terrier, Daisy, has died. 'I couldn't bear to see her suffer,' she says, simply. 'She'd had cancer and was so ill. She just wasn't having fun anymore. Her little doggy life really wasn't worth living.'

She goes on to tell me how the vet came to her cottage and Daisy was injected while lying in her favourite chair, my friend stroking her all the while. 'She was gone in seconds. I am heartbroken,' she admits, 'but so relieved she went that way, and she didn't have to feel any more pain. My neighbours joined me to celebrate her life with a glass of champagne.'

I so wish we could do the same for James and Bonnie when the time comes. Our society is more compassionate to animals than it is to its people.

John reminds me that the worst is yet to come. How could it be?

He is right, as it happens. Things are getting worse. Bonnie has broken her hip. I can only imagine how the visit to the local hospital and the pain she was feeling must have frightened her. John is distraught. How do you explain to a dementia patient that she is going to need a hip replacement?

I go with John to the hospital. She's looking weak and fragile, the skin on her face transparent. She is totally unaware of our presence. She cries out when the carers try to lift her out of the chair for the physiotherapist to walk her, so they give up, abandoning the idea of taking even a few steps. In her chair she wriggles in discomfort. We ask, 'Do you think Bonnie needs some pain relief?'

A young nurse asks, 'Bonnie, are you in pain?'

John explodes, 'How the hell can Bonnie possibly answer your question? She has dementia for Christ's sake! How can she tell you?'

I'm feeling no less furious and frustrated, as much with myself as with the care home doctor. He gives James course after course of antibiotics for his dental abscesses, but when a dentist is finally called to see him it is clear she is shocked.

'Why haven't we seen James before this? He's got a loose bridge and seems to have had several abscesses, as well as exposed nerves. Poor chap must be in terrible pain. We'll need a hospital appointment as soon as possible.'

It seems that James needs his teeth removed under general anaesthetic but I am warned that waiting lists are lengthy. Oh God, why did we let it come to this? Why didn't I take control of the situation earlier? I'd accepted a carer's reassurance, who told me, 'It's normal for dementia patients to get dental problems, it's impossible to clean their teeth and they don't know the difference between a mouthwash and a drink, and what's more they don't even feel pain.' My instincts told me otherwise, yet I didn't argue.

The doctor continues to dole out antibiotics and Panadol. I remember James's and my pact. We promised each other that we'd do everything possible to put the other one out of their misery should we ever become so ill or incapacitated that life isn't worth living. How simple the words seemed then, so easy to say. Now I wish I had the courage to put a pillow over his head. But I don't, even though watching all this unroll has become the stuff of nightmares.

James and Bonnie share a list of 'nevers'. They will:

never know us again;

never travel abroad again;

never see Paris again;

never kiss again;

never make love again;

never have lovely chats again;

never laugh out loud again;

never enjoy a glass of champagne again;

never enjoy a gourmet meal again;

never enjoy a film again;

never play chess again ;

never do the crossword again;

never sail in a boat again;

never drive a car again;

never sing again;

never read a book again;

never have fun again;

never swim in the sea again;

never know their family again;

never know who they were again;

never know life again;

never have a conversation again.

Sometimes the weight of knowing that they are sentenced to a non-life makes John and myself even more aware of the life we have, and how we have a duty to make the best of it. Dementia has taken so much, we don't want to let it take everything – we can't let the bastard D win.

* * *

I visit Germany with John. He's researching his book on Beethoven, his hero, and not for the first time am I reminded of my wandering around Vienna with James while he was writing about Mozart, whom he similarly adored. These strange parallels and similarities comfort me.

We sit in the pretty town square of Rüdesheim on the Rhine, soaking up the sunshine and drinking the local wine. We share our memories of our various youthful visits to Germany and laugh together.

'I was seventeen. On a school trip,' John remembers. 'I was very proud of my German, my best subject. There was a redhead I fell in love with. It was a cruel blow to my self-esteem when she didn't respond to my schoolboy advances.' Laughing, he shrugs his shoulders. 'But I got over it.'

I remember James telling me a very similar story. He had spent three months studying German on a student exchange and he'd fallen in love with a beautiful, blonde local girl.

They wrote to each other for a year but when she came to England she fell in love with another boy and left James with a broken heart.

I tell John how I'd hitchhiked around Europe as an eighteen-year-old student, staying in youth hostels. In Munich, a young man offered to help me and my friends find our hostel and he invited us to have supper with his family. Next day he gave us a tour of the city and gave me a small bottle of Nina Ricci's L'Air du Temps perfume, making me promise I'd see him again. My friends, who like me could never have afforded to buy the perfume for themselves, joked that he must have stolen it from his mother. He wrote to me afterwards but I soon lost interest, although I did fall in love with the Nina Ricci, and still wear it to this day.

It feels good laughing about our youthful exploits. James's story has its place at the table, which seems only right as he's not here to tell it himself.

* * *

I want to tell James that I saw the first swallows of the year yesterday, but he's in his bed asleep and I'm sitting in a chair beside him. I gaze at the photograph, on his wall, of the five fledglings on a beam in our old barn, and am reminded of how much he loved these small precision-flying birds that spend most of their time on the wing, aerial feeding. James used to describe them as 'Spitfires in the sky' that had flown bravely all the way from Africa.

Generations of swallows raised their young in the barn year after year. James photographed their progress from the moment they arrived and built their nests. I will never forget the joy on his face the day we watched the young fledglings lining up one by one on the beam, preparing to fly for the first time.

He's woken now. I lean close to him so that he can smell my perfume, a scent he loved. He looks at me when I take his hand and his eyes blink, trying to focus. He stares into my face for a long time as a I whisper loving words. Is there any recognition? I'm not sure. I stroke his hair and face, and kiss him gently on the cheek. I hold my face close to allow him time to recognise me, but I get no reaction. Instead he looks away and out beyond me into the room.

It's strange that with all the physical ravages dementia has wrought, it has left James's beautiful hands untouched. Strangely, they haven't aged. I rub hand cream into them and trim his nails.

I can see him now, talking with his hands. He always gesticulated as he told a story, and it was wonderfully expressive. It was one of the first things I noticed about him. James always loved food, believing, quite rightly, that it is an extension of love. He'd gather all the herbs and spices together to make a perfect curry or pasta, creating gorgeous aromas in the kitchen. 'Love and food go together,' he'd say.

James had no time for faddy diets, or for women who didn't love their food. I can still hear him say, 'Give me a fleshy woman any day. They're so much sexier.'

Alice, a carer, gives me a tray with James's lunch. It's a bowl of brown goo.

'What is it?'

She answers cheerily, 'Mashed potato and vegetable soup.'

It takes an age to feed him. He opens his mouth only when I part his lips with the spoon. He's like a fledgling bird, and yet unlike a fledgling he takes no interest in eating.

He falls asleep and I look out on my life.

I have a long bucket list of places I've always wanted to visit and experience life there. I'd like to take a train across Canada; to learn the tango, as it should be danced, in the bars of Buenos Aires; to watch the whales in Akureyri; to sail around the Norwegian fjords; to visit the Galapagos islands or stand atop the ancient wonder of Machu Picchu; to travel across Siberia by train to Beijing, or visit Kerala on the Arabian Sea where the pace of life seems to be as languid as its backwaters.

I want to get back to my art. To sculpt and paint in my own studio.

I have no energy for any of it. I've sunk so low.

I look at James sleeping. I can hear him saying, 'Get out there and do it.'

* * *

Even away from the care home, dementia always plonks itself into the middle of our evening. John and I talk about James and Bonnie over supper and it's strange that here we are, continuing to care for two people who haven't spoken or acknowledged either one of us for nigh on ten years.

John asks me to renovate his flat on the river, knowing it will do me good having a project to get my teeth into. He allows me a complete say in everything, and I choose all the furniture, bed linen, kitchenware and lamps, and redesign the layout. It works like a dream, opening out spaces and creating more storage. It is springtime, and I feel compelled to bring as much air and light into the apartment as I can. I replace the heavy curtains at the windows of the large open-plan living room with shutters painted into the wall, and hang mirrors in all the dark areas, which now reflect the light and bring in the river.

The loveliest thing in the whole room, and around which I plan the colour scheme, is a pale aqua rug that John and Bonnie had bought together.

* * *

We go to Sicily in August, to a lovely old villa belonging to a friend, that sits on the edge of the Mediterranean. We have the beach to ourselves.

Every day after breakfast we sit out on the terrace in the

garden and read our books or listen to music. Later in the morning we walk the length of the sandy white beach and afterwards, hot and sweaty, we plunge into the cool, azure sea for a swim. We drink wine at lunchtime and doze in the afternoon.

I think about James and how he would love it here in the sun; his lithe and perfect body would always turn the colour of caramel in a matter of days.

Sadness and guilt cling to me for the rest of the day. In the evening John notices my pensive mood and asks me to please come back to him. But it's no good. I can't shift it.

21 : Kinder to Animals

It's not that I loved you less
Than when at your feet I lay:
But to prevent the sad increase
Of hopeless love, I keep away
*   — Edmund Waller*

Soon after our return from Sicily I need to take James to the dental clinic. I am startled to see the effect the short taxi ride has on him. He is visibly terrified. People and traffic are moving too fast for him. He starts to shake.

At the clinic they only say the same thing they've said before – that he urgently needs his teeth removed under general anaesthetic. James sits helplessly in his wheelchair, feeling bewildered and under attack, as the dentist tries to insert metal instruments into his mouth.

I'm furious. 'Why hasn't he been given an appointment to get the work done? I've heard all this before.'

She apologises. 'I'm very sorry. We must have lost him in the system. I can't find any trace of his notes.'

On the way back to the care home James is sick all over his clothes, the seat, and the floor of the taxi. The driver is furious, ranting and shouting at me, and I give him an extra twenty after I try to sort out James.

Things go from bad to worse. The day of his surgery I get him to the hospital only to find that the ambulance has brought us to the wrong place. By the time I get the consultant on the phone she says that it's too late to operate on James – it's a day centre apparently, which closes at seven.

'Unfortunately, the next available appointment for a surgery like this isn't for another two months.'

Angry and defeated I fall on his chair in tears. I wheel James back downstairs to wait for the ambulance. By now the sedation has worn off and he is completely alert. The return journey is a nightmare; terrified, he becomes violently sick again and covers both of us in vomit. Then he soils himself and diarrhoea and urine escape his incontinence pad and stream down his trouser legs, filling his shoes and pooling onto the floor of the ambulance.

I sit with my arms around him, the situation sending me into a spiral of rage.

I curse the hospital's mix-up;

I curse the care home's incompetence;

I curse the ambulance service.;

And, most of all, I curse bloody dementia.

The bastard Dementia is out to get me too. I collapse a few days later with the worst chest infection ever. It takes me several weeks to recover after three lots of antibiotics and a course of steroids....

I notice James's swallow reflex is going. It's taken me over an hour to feed him a teaspoon of mashed banana and yogurt. I wrap my arms around him and we sit in silence while our old photographs stare down on us like ghosts.

As I am leaving, a woman who'd been visiting her mother comes over to me and whispers, 'It's heartbreaking isn't it? We're kinder to animals.' I nod. I don't need reminding.

It's only on the train back to London that I realise I haven't had anything to eat or drink all day. Back at the flat, John gives me a hug. Unable to talk, I sob. He makes me a cup of tea. I make a fish pie, hoping it will distract me from the sadness of the day. It doesn't, and the glass of wine John pours me also fails to lift my mood.

John chats away about his day, finally saying, 'Did you hear any of that? You're not listening.'

I can't engage, nor can I eat a mouthful of the food I'd prepared. Eventually I fall into bed, our evening ruined, having drunk too much wine on an empty stomach.

* * *

We visit Verona to see *La Traviata*. I remember going to the amphitheatre with James after he'd been diagnosed. First he'd refused to remove his sunhat, then the emotion of *La Bohème* had been too much for him and he'd broken down in tears and sobbed like a baby. The audience had watched us, incredulous. Some were visibly annoyed; others tittered, assuming he was an eccentric.

Now I find myself enjoying every bit of the opera. This time it is me who cries silent tears. I cry for James and Bonnie and their lost lives. I cry for Violetta, and I cry for me. The tears are a mixture of sadness and joy.

I am alive. I'm listening to the most beautiful music in the most spectacular place, with a man who is giving me a reason to live again.

We finish our evening dining out in the piazza with a glass of Chianti. This time we drink to 'John and Nula.'

* * *

There's a heatwave when we return. I find James out in the garden, in his special chair. I laugh when I see him dressed in a pair of shorts, a straw sun hat, red socks and slippers, none of them his. He's fast asleep. I laugh with the carers. Lighter moments like this are becoming increasingly rare.

When he eventually opens his eyes I kneel down in front of him, lean across and stroke his cheek. I hold my face close, saying, 'Jamesie, Jamesie, it's me.' I say it again, gently kissing his cheek. He blinks his eyes and looks through me. His lips move as if he's trying to say something, then I get the biggest smile.

I am so happy with the smile, thinking there's been a window of recognition. But then I'm jolted back to reality when a carer comes over to his chair and gets exactly the same reaction from him.

* * *

John and I visit Aix-en-Provence. Years before, James and I had stayed there while he filmed a series on France, Trading Places. He'd loved Provence and planned one day to buy an old house we could renovate, in the hills above Nice, far away from tourists. I'd envisioned a blonde stone villa with pale eau de nil painted shutters, looking out onto a large terraced garden full of lavender, drinking our rosé wine, a view of the Mediterranean in the distance. In our retirement, James would write and, as the colours and light of Provence beg to be put on canvas, I would paint.

I tell John how James used to tease me, saying, 'If anything happens to me, I'd still want you to go and live there, find a handsome French man and live happily ever after.'

John says, 'Will I do? I speak French.'

* * *

On my return from France, I find James has deteriorated dreadfully. The care home manager says that she thinks he is near the end and that the doctor has made an appointment for him to be seen by the palliative care team.

I believe them all when I'm told they will ensure his end is as pain-free and comfortable as possible when the time comes.

Just when I need it most there is a moment of recognition, a little crack in that seemingly closed window. I'm sitting next to James's bed, holding his hands. I press my face onto his cheek so he can feel my warmth. Then he holds my stare and we connect. Yes, yes, yes, I am certain of it – a definite connection. Oh my God, I can't believe it! It brings back something I heard as a child growing up in rural Ireland: that when someone is near to death they get a momentary awareness. Is this true?

I scrabble in my handbag for my earphones. I put them into James's ears and play his favourite Mozart. He reacts to it immediately and his eyes fill with tears that slowly trickle down his cheeks. I then put on the old Irish folksong – The Isle of Innisfree, 'But dreams don't last / Though dreams are not forgotten, / … / I still would choose the isle of Innisfree'. We'd always loved the words – being Irish ourselves – which tell of an Irish immigrant longing for his homeland. Again I get the same reaction.

It feels like an intermittent beacon illuminating our shared history and enduring love. For the first time in years we are united by the music, and it is as if James is saying goodbye with all his love. I hug him and hug him and kiss away his tears.

* * *

Palliative care, as it turns out, was not a team, just one nurse. It's a misnomer when it comes to James's treatment. Whenever it is clear he is feeling pain, such as those times he is hoisted in and out of bed, I am told by the palliative care nurse that, 'dementia patients don't feel pain'. This is followed by the assurance that after the procedure, 'He'll forget very quickly anyway.'

Bloody hell, this is not palliative care!

In the days that follow, his condition fluctuates. He rebounds for a short while and he has a shower, smiles and eats his food, and I'm almost fooled that he's on the mend. He's done this a few times. Then afterwards he deteriorates further. But I know that it is bloody dementia playing its dirty tricks on me and it won't last. My instincts are that James's life is ebbing away. He has no strength to fight anymore.

* * *

I'm in the supermarket with a trolley full of shopping when I get the call: 'Come as soon as you can. James isn't going to make it.'

I abandon the trolley and run to the station. In my distress I get on the wrong train. A young police officer notices me looking frantic and in tears.

'Are you okay? Are you lost?'

She accompanies me to the right platform and remains with me until I'm on the train. She is an angel.

When I arrive at the care home James is shaking violently. These fits, Dee his carer tells me, are a sign his body is shutting down, unable to cope. He's been given course after course of antibiotics for his diarrhoea, and I am filled with a fury that it's all been pointless – that what he's really needing is someone kindly to ease his discomfort.

When I ask the doctor to do something, please, to ease his suffering, he looks at me, aghast.

'Are you asking me to murder him?'

He tells me James hasn't yet reached the critical stage and that we have to wait to let it happen naturally, 'in God's own good time'. I could hit him. I'd fallen out with God a long time ago – I'd seen too many injustices happen to the loveliest people for no reason.

One of the nurses tells me that Harold Shipman, the serial killer doctor, has a lot to answer for. Apparently, since his trial, rules around palliative care have been tightened, to the extent that some doctors no longer feel able to administer morphine in the kind of compassionate doses poor souls like James require.

* * *

I stay with James for several days and nights. Sitting in a

chair close to his bed I reminisce on our old life. The events that led to our meeting on location in Africa. Our life together. The happiness and fun he brought me. The way he saw life in a totally positive way. There was no such word as 'No' in his vocabulary. I thought of all the 'what might have beens'.

* * *

I can't eat or sleep. Finally, beaten down, I return to John's flat.

He tries to comfort and hug me but I push him away. My emotions are anaesthetised. I am unable to speak.

I feel nauseous. He pours me a large brandy. I fall into bed but am unable to sleep. I get up and go into the study, from where I call the care home every hour through the night. I'm told to please, please stop calling – that I need to take care of myself, that I should sleep. The night nurse tells me that if there's the slightest change she will call.

At seven a.m. there's a call. 'I think you should come as soon as you can. James has deteriorated hugely in the last hour.'

* * *

I watch him struggle to breathe. His ribcage looks as though it's going to break through the transparent skin of his chest.

He plucks the bedclothes in anxiety. The morphine patch prescribed by the doctor is woefully inadequate. How can I endure watching him suffer like this?

But James lingers on. While I am trying to cope with this, inevitably my relationship with John suffers. He's trying to 'be there for me', attempting to comfort me, but I refuse all his efforts to console me.

'I'm sure James won't last too long. His suffering will be over soon.'

I'm not in the right frame of mind to hear his words.

He continues, refusing to give up. 'I'll be with you all the way. When it does happen, I'll be there. I'll never let you go.'

He tries to distract me by taking me out to dinner, knowing I've hardly eaten anything for the past week. I try to eat, but the food is like sawdust in my mouth. I can't respond to his chat either. I can tell he's upset. We return home and ignore each other for the rest of the evening.

* * *

It's a week after James's crisis, and this time John's upset over Bonnie. He went to the care home to find her slumped in a chair with her head bowed to her chest. She was agitated, rubbing her head constantly with her hand.

The carer asks Bonnie, 'Is your head hurting?', which caused John to erupt: 'For God's sake, Bon has dementia.

She can't understand.'

Embarrassed, she rushed off to find some Panadol.

We're unable to comfort each other. Dementia dominates our chat, and the atmosphere is full of anxiety. We're helpless in relieving either James's or Bonnie's suffering.

John persists patiently in trying to talk to me but I am indifferent. 'We're in this together, Nuli. Whatever happens to James or Bonnie – when it's their turn to go – we'll be there to comfort and love each other through it.'

I'm not so sure I can do this: love in the present when you're grieving in the past. I want to get as far away as possible from dementia – and John.

But he is insistent and holds me tight. 'Please, please don't push me away. Don't let bloody dementia win!'

'It's already won. We're unable to give James and Bonnie any words of comfort. We can't even say goodbye,' I said, raving like a lunatic. 'And as for us, it's smashing us too.'

Next evening John sits me down. 'We have to support each other through this,' he said patiently. 'And not only that. You have to be strong, not only for your sake, but for James's too. You're the only one who can fight his corner.'

I know he's right.

* * *

I try to be strong but in the weeks that follow, James's condition descends into a nightmare cycle of crisis after crisis. It's inevitable after six weeks of chronic diarrhoea caused by a C Difficile infection, and the four lots of drugs prescribed to halt it that did not work, coupled with his inability to eat, that he has suffered a massive weight loss. He looks skeletal and cries out each time the carers remove his soiled incontinence pads. The constant changing of the pads and his extreme weight loss have caused chronic bedsores on his buttocks, knees and hip bones. Eventually he's so weak that even the effort to cry out is too much for him.

I am horrified to discover that even at this stage not one member of staff – the doctor, care home manager, palliative care nurse (with the exception of one carer) – discussed with me James's condition and end of life. No one prepared me for how intolerable the final days would be. And never in my most awful nightmares could I have imagined such a terrible ending to a human life.

In desperation I ring a hospice in Cambridge to plead with them to take James. They ask what his condition is. I said he had end stage dementia. 'Sorry,' they say, 'but we can't take him, because dementia patients take a long time to die and we can't evaluate how long that might be, and we have so many terminal cancer patients to care for who have only weeks or days to live.'

Finally I lose control and scream at the care home staff. 'Please, please call a doctor immediately!'

They try to calm me, to reassure me that James probably

isn't aware, and I shout at them that he bloody well is.

The doctor arrives several hours later and looks visibly shocked when he sees James. He admits that his deterioration is beyond what he'd expected when he'd seen him four days ago.

Fighting back my tears, I said, 'Dr ... Maybe you can show some compassion now. Why did you allow him to suffer so long?'

I accuse him of doing dying by the book and having no compassion.

With embarrassment in his voice, he says, 'It wasn't easy to gauge, James was difficult, he kept fighting back.'

Furious I ask, 'Do you really think looking at the state of him he was in any fit state to fight back?'

He immediately increases the morphine for the pain, and medazalem to ease James's anxiety.

* * *

I don't leave James's bedside for the next few weeks. In the long bleak hours of the final days, as death creeps closer to him, I stroke his hair and tell him how much I love him and will never stop loving him. I long to keep him beside me but know death demands that he undertakes this journey without me, however often I promise to look after him and protect him. I must relinquish him to be free from this dreaded disease.

He moves in and out of consciousness and, constantly vigilant, unable to sleep, exhausted after several days and nights, I am finally persuaded to go home and get some rest. I shower at John's flat, and take a sleeping pill, planning to go straight back in the morning.

But the bastard D takes James in my absence.

At 6:15 the telephone wakes me. 'It's the night nurse here, Nula. I'm sorry to tell you James has just passed away. His sister Angela was with him. It was very peaceful.'

No, no, no, I sob down the telephone. The nurse tells me gently, 'Sometimes they don't want you there. Maybe your not being there allowed him to leave.'

* * *

When I enter James's room I'm struck by the eerie silence. Everything is as before – the same photos look down on him from the walls –

I fall on him and cover his face with mine. 'Jamesie, my Jamesie, my Jamesie!' I howl.

Dee – our beloved carer who had come in on her day off to be with me – has dressed him in a suit he had worn so many times to glamorous events and that once had made him look so stunningly handsome. Now it only emphasises his emaciated body invaded by the dreaded dementia.

I sit alone with his ravaged body. The silent room enshrouds us.

I put a few little things into the pockets of his suit: pictures of his beloved corgi, Spanny; a favourite salmon-fishing fly; some photographs, and a personal note from me. I spray my perfume on him.

Dee interrupts and whispers, 'The undertakers are here.'

Sobbing, I kiss him. I cannot say goodbye, it means going away for ever. The thought of never seeing him again overwhelms me.

22 : Final Goodbyes

We must let go of the life we have planned, so as to accept the one that is waiting for us – Joseph Campbell

Two weeks later James is cremated. It is a simple, humanitarian farewell ceremony, as was his wish. The day is mild but overcast. Then it starts to drizzle. The light rain reminds me of what James always said on a day like this: 'Perfect weather for fly fishing.' I smile inside at the thought.

The awful moment when the hearse rounds the corner is lightened slightly by a tall, striking young woman in top hat and tails, wielding an umbrella, walking in front of the vehicle. James would have liked that.

We followed his coffin into the chapel to Mozart's *Ave Verum Corpus*. We say our last goodbyes to this Belfast boy, with a tenor singing his dearly loved 'Londonderry Air', that James sang at so many parties. The celebrant reads his favourite W.B. Yeats poem, 'The Lake Isle of Innisfree'

I will arise and go now, and go to Innisfree,
And a small cabin build there, of clay and wattles made;
Nine bean-rows will I have there, a hive for the honey-bee,

And live alone in the bee-loud glade.
And I shall have some peace there, for peace comes
    dropping slow

Dropping from the veils of the morning to where the
    cricket sings;
There midnight's all a glimmer, and noon a purple glow,
And evening full of the linnet's wings.

I will arise and go now, for always night and day
I hear lake water lapping with low sounds by the shore;
While I stand on the roadway, or on the pavements grey,
I hear it in the deep heart's core.

* * *

Three months after James's funeral I get one of my dear wishes: John and I travel to India and visit Kerala. It is everything I'd hoped for, a harmonious rainbow of colours. We stay in a fisherman's hut on the edge of a golden beach. It is so tranquil. Our cottage is called Moksha, meaning Freedom.

Kerala has a spirituality about it that wraps itself around me. In this healing place I think a lot about the past, trying to find a meaning in the pain and sadness of the last years and months.

In the early evenings we sit out on our terrace and watch the sunset. After ten days I slip into a peace I haven't felt in a long, long time.

* * *

Five months later it is Bonnie's time to go. I am happy that she is in the caring and compassionate hands of an 'old school' doctor, a man who has practised medicine for over thirty years. He administers the best pain and anxiety relief possible and makes sure that her dying is as quick, calm and peaceful as it could be. That is a huge comfort to John and her two sons who were with her till the end.

She, too, has a simple humanitarian service. So soon after losing James, I find it especially hard reliving all the emotions again. John and I break down at the sight of Bonnie's coffin and we hug each other.

The closing music at her funeral service is Joan Baez's 'Farewell Angelina' – a much-loved favourite of Bonnie's – and strangely the first LP I ever bought as a student. It strikes me that this gives me a connection to her even after death.

* * *

In the weeks that follow I'm hit by an overwhelming tsunami of sadness. I can't understand why. It is all over. James and Bonnie are free.

In the months after James's death the agony of loss pervades, it's unbearable. Outside he is gone but inside he's infinitely present. I cry for days and cannot lift the darkness that hangs over me. I try to find a magic recipe to conquer the heartache but there is nothing to ease the pain. I have no choice but to give in to the grief. I replay over and over again all the happy memories, times, chats, and journeys we shared. I absorb all the feelings and allow the sadness to envelope me. I can't find any peace. I want to run far away from John and all the reminders of dementia.

A month after Bonnie's funeral I decide to leave John. I return to my flat outside London and attempt to gain a little space and time to sort myself out. The years of battling and surviving have taken their toll. My grieving mind is jumping into strange patterns of thinking. I am not the same person. I need to find myself and forge a new road forward.

I have decided our relationship is over. It had been a challenging journey, with rocky moments as well as interludes of utter joy. Dementia brought us together, now there is no need for us to stay that way. When I put it to John, he agrees. He has been thinking the same way. Our relationship has run its course.

But over the next days and weeks he continues to text and e-mail me — nothing intimate, just things he's read in the papers, musical events, new films released. Then he remembers we have an appointment at the Apple Store to sort my computer out. He says we shouldn't let it go — we had to wait long enough to get it. So we meet up again.

We have lunch afterwards in Covent Garden. We talk and talk and talk. I look at him across the table. How could

I ever think of leaving this man? Has he not taken me from the depths of hopelessness to somewhere different, the next step towards recovery? Has he not been my rock these past months? Has grief not proved to me how fragile and precious life is?

We have gone through so much together in the years of tragic and heartbreaking dementia; shared so much pain and sadness. Our lives are intertwined. He's come to know me in these past years like no-one else, at my lowest, and understands and loves all my foibles. Our initial bond was dementia. He lost Bonnie and I lost James; he understands things that other people don't. We have each taken each other to different places from where we were when we first met. I cannot now imagine my life without him.

Surely it was okay to begin a new journey with him by my side?

I love him for Christ's sake.

After the lunch, we get a rickshaw ride to the station and laugh at the craziness of it all. Yes, life beckons. We need to grasp it and make the most of the time we have left. For the first time in weeks we hug.

* * *

The ashes of Bonnie and James lie beside each other for several weeks in John's flat. In a strange way it's a huge comfort to have the four of us together.

Some months later we take Bonnie's ashes to her favourite park. We stand with her two sons, her daughter-in-law, and her two adorable grandchildren and scatter them in a rose garden, at the roots of a rosebush that is aptly named 'Lovely Lady'.

I decide to put some of James's ashes with Bonnie. They had shared a corridor and a journey for nigh on six years. The remainder I take, with his sister Maureen and brother Peter, to Belfast. It is an emotional journey. I insist we drive through his past: the old streets that were his playground; the home where they all grew up; his grammar school.

We unite James with his adored grandmother and his parents.

That evening, in a local hotel, over dinner we laugh and cry at our shared memories. It is what James would have wished. We drink to him and agree how lucky we've been to have had him in our lives.

23 : Making a New Life

Across the gateway of my heart I wrote
'No thoroughfare'
But love came laughing by,
And cried I enter everywhere.
                              – Herbert Shipman

James and Bonnie, our lives with them, and their love have left their imprints everywhere. When you lose someone so close to you they're always there, and it's impossible not to carry a piece of them with you. I hear myself asking James for advice in moments of stress. It's impossible not to be reminded of him and our life together – a flower, a moment, a piece of music, a film and think how much he would have loved this or that.

The tears fall for his lost life and my love for him will never die. John does exactly the same thing as memories of his life with Bonnie surface. We include them in our conversations. When talking about the past John will say, when Bonnie and I went here or there or did such and such. I do exactly the same. They will always be part of our lives we will never ever forget them.

We agree on one thing: death does not consume love;

that loves survives, its branches spreading; renewing and replenishing, that for now, to love and be loved is all that matters.

My journey to this happy place has taken a long time, but what I have learned more than anything is the wonderful revelation that I am in charge of my own life, and in charge of what I choose to do with it. Perhaps the biggest surprise of all is that it is possible, at any age and any time, to find someone to cherish and to love.

* * *

In 2016 we decide to return to India. Just as we settle into our flight John turns to me, smiling. 'I have something to ask you. Will you marry me?'

My eyes fill up with tears, and an air stewardess passing our seats asks, 'Are you okay?'

John laughs and says, 'I've just proposed to her. She said yes.' She returns with two glasses of champagne.

John chooses the seventh day of the seventh month for our wedding, because he knows seven is my lucky number. We marry in the East End of London with just a few close family and friends there.

* * *

In September, John's new book, Mozart, the Man Revealed,

is published. He dedicates it to the memory of 'Mozart lover James Black'.

Finally I feel a return of creative energy, feeling it rising up like sap in me after a decade of flat hopelessness. I've changed as a person. The loss of James has made me see life in a different way. I'm a bigger, better person because of it. My life now, once again, is about love.

Postscript

Dementia is in the news – constantly. Not a day goes by when there's not a story in the papers on some aspect of the disease, whether it is to do with research, lack of care, scarcity of resources, or most often some way of behaving that will lessen your chances of developing it.

You never see the most truthful story of all, which would say: 'Whether you develop dementia or not is down to a roll of the dice. You are lucky or unlucky. If you are unlucky, expect no cure, no effective treatment, no specialist care, with very little help for those caring for you.'

Here are a selection of recent dementia headlines in the papers:

Third of dying patients 'are given needless treatments'.

Doctors and nurses 'walk on by' as patients are dying'.

Dementia patients charged up to 40% extra by care homes.

Dementia patients left in agony as they can't explain their pain to nurses.

Dementia patients in care homes 'are 2nd-class citizens'.

Dementia Betrayal: Half of NHS trusts providing poor care and hundreds and thousands not diagnosed.

They wouldn't say that about cancer, would they? And yet dementia has overtaken cancer, heart disease, and stroke as the biggest killer in the UK.

So you would expect money to be thrown at research into finding a cure for this mass killer. But an Oxford University study showed that dementia receives a fraction of the sum allocated to cancer and heart disease. There are over 1,000 new drugs in the pipeline for cancer. There are 80 in the pipeline for dementia. The NHS boasts some of the finest cancer specialists in the world. Those in care homes with dementia are treated by GPs.

Why does this woeful state of affairs go unnoticed by those in power? The short answer is that it doesn't. In 2015 John and I met the then Secretary of State for Health Jeremy Hunt to discuss government plans to put dementia at the forefront of health policy. How? By improving diagnosis. Our plea to train more dementia specialists and improve care home skills was met with a serious nod, but diagnosis comes first. John was told he would be put on a panel to look at ways of improving dementia care. We never heard another word after that.

Dementia patients are currently charged around 15%

more for care because they are considered harder to look after. When this became known, a cross-party group of MPs demanded that more money should be made available to the NHS to cover these extra costs. I suggest you don't hold your breath.

On average GPs spend ten minutes visiting dementia patients in care homes. Ten minutes? This is woefully inadequate. Without doubt dementia sufferers are hugely neglected. Dementia is a terminal disease, and those with it should be given the same support as someone with cancer. I witnessed myself how some care home managers and GPs actually refused to visit patients, particularly out of hours.

The most effective campaign on behalf of those with dementia and their carers comes from well-known figures who speak out about it. In 2019 the actress Vicky McClure (from TV's Line of Duty) presented a wonderful two-part television programme bringing together those with dementia to form a choir and give a public performance on the stage of Nottingham's Royal Concert Hall. One TV critic said Vicky had done more for dementia in two hours than politicians had in years.

When former Formula One champion Jackie Stewart went public about his wife Helen's dementia, saying he was devoting his life to helping to find a cure by launching a £2 million fund for research, he increased awareness of dementia more than any government, or report, or statistic ever can.

A cure for dementia is a long way off, we all know that. But conditions for those with dementia and their carers could be improved immeasurably with a single signature on a piece of paper.

The worst part for me was the lack of palliative care. Early palliative care would greatly improve the quality of life for patients and their families, and give people an honest conversation about treatment and what to expect as their condition worsens. This would make harmful intervention at the end of a loved one's life less likely, and help families prepare for the inevitable end.

As things stand, there is little care for people with dementia, and even less for those caring for them. It is time the NHS addressed the problem head on. Otherwise dementia will overwhelm us, as well as the NHS we are so proud of.

Above all, I want to see people like me given the right to choose at what point their loved should be allowed to die with dignity, and overrule a GP like the one I encountered who accused me of asking him to play God.

All of this is why I felt compelled to write this book.

Acknowledgements

I want to thank my dearest friend Colette Coyle who stood by me through it all. She knew and adored James from the very beginning and it was her constant love and support that kept us going especially in the first stages of the dementia journey. She made sure she was with me when I made the horrible journey with him to the care home. She was always on hand when I fell apart and ready with a hug, a delicious meal and a glass of wine. Anything to encourage me to continue with my life.

Mona Guckian-Fisher, who out of the blue wrote to John when he was supporting Dementia UK, to say she was a health care professional, and was caring for her husband, who had dementia. She was appalled at the lack of support for people looking after those with dementia, and had written to the then Prime Minister David Cameron outlining her concerns. We have since come to know Mona well, count her among our dearest friends, and will for ever be grateful for the support she gave John and me when we were going through our dementia crisis. Mona's husband Phil, a head teacher, was diagnosed with dementia at the age of 51, and died twelve years later. This book is dedicated to our three spouses, James, Bonnie and Phil, whom Mona has christened The Trinity.

Dee Tibbles, a very special carer who went above and beyond her duties to give James the best care, and was with me through the whole final journey. Even afterwards she helped me deal with the formalities of death certificate and undertakers, and she and her family were there to support me at the funeral.

Author Note

Nula Suchet was born and raised in Ireland, part of a large family. She studied Art and Design at Chelsea College of Art and became an interior designer, working internationally in the UK, Europe and the US. Now retired, she lives in London with her husband, the broadcaster John Suchet.